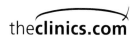

CLINICS IN
SPORTS MEDICINE

Foot and Ankle Injuries in Dance

GUEST EDITORS
John G. Kennedy, MD
Christopher W. Hodgkins, MD

CONSULTING EDITOR
Mark D. Miller, MD

April 2008 • Volume 27 • Number 2

SAUNDERS

An Imprint of Elsevier, Inc.
PHILADELPHIA   LONDON   TORONTO   MONTREAL   SYDNEY   TOKYO

W.B. SAUNDERS COMPANY
A Division of Elsevier Inc.

1600 John F. Kennedy Blvd. • Suite 1800 • Philadelphia, Pennsylvania 19103

http://www.theclinics.com

CLINICS IN SPORTS MEDICINE	**Volume 27, Number 2**
April 2008	**ISSN 0278-5919**
Editor: Debora Dellapena	**ISBN-13: 978-1-4160-5811-3**
	ISBN-10: 1-4160-5811-7

Reprints: For copies of 100 or more, of articles in this publication, please contact the Commercial Reprints Department, Elsevier Inc., 360 Park Avenue South, New York, New York 10010-1710. Tel. (212) 633-3813; Fax: (212) 462-1935 e-mail: reprints@elsevier.com.

The ideas and opinions expressed in *Clinics in Sports Medicine* do not necessarily reflect those of the Publisher. The Publisher does not assume any responsibility for any injury and/or damage to persons or property arising out of or related to any use of the material contained in this periodical. The reader is advised to check the appropriate medical literature and the product information currently provided by the manufacturer of each drug to be administered to verify the dosage, the method and duration of administration, or contraindications. It is the responsibility of the treating physician or other health care professional, relying on independent experience and knowledge of the patient, to determine drug dosages and the best treatment for the patient. Mention of any product in this issue should not be construed as endorsement by the contributors, editors, or the Publisher of the product or manufacturers' claims.

Clinics in Sports Medicine (ISSN 0278-5919) is published quarterly by Elsevier Inc., 360 Park Avenue South, New York, NY 10010-1710. Months of publication are January, April, July, and October. Business and Editorial Offices: 1600 John F. Kennedy Blvd., Suite 1800, Philadelphia, PA 19103-2899. Customer Service Offices: 6277 Sea Harbor Drive, Orlando, FL 32887-4800. Periodicals postage paid at New York, NY, and additional mailing offices. Subscription prices are $230.00 per year (US individuals), $357.00 per year (US institutions), $115.00 per year (US students), $260.00 per year (Canadian individuals), $423.00 per year (Canadian institutions), $151.00 (Canadian students), $297.00 per year (foreign individuals), $423.00 per year (foreign institutions), and $151.00 per year (foreign students). Foreign air speed delivery is included in all *Clinics* subscription prices. All prices are subject to change without notice. POSTMASTER: Send address changes to *Clinics in Sports Medicine*, Elsevier Periodicals Customer Service, 6277 Sea Harbor Drive, Orlando, FL 32887-4800. Customer Service: 1-800-654-2452 (US). From outside the United States, call 1-407-563-6020. Fax: 1-407-363-9661. E-mail: JournalsCustomerService-usa@elsevier.com.

Clinics in Sports Medicine is covered in *Index Medicus, Current Contents/Clinical Medicine, Excerpta Medica,* and *ISI/Biomed.*

Printed in the United States of America.

ELSEVIER
SAUNDERS

CLINICS IN SPORTS MEDICINE

Foot and Ankle Injuries in Dance

CONSULTING EDITOR

MARK D. MILLER, MD, Professor, Department of Orthopaedic Surgery; Head, Division of Sports Medicine, University of Virginia Health System, Charlottesville, Virginia

GUEST EDITORS

JOHN G. KENNEDY, MD, MMSc, MCh, FRCSI, FRCS (Orth), Assistant Professor of Orthopaedic Surgery, Hospital for Special Surgery, New York, New York

CHRISTOPHER W. HODGKINS, MD, Orthopaedic Surgery Resident, Department of Orthopaedic Surgery, University of Miami, Miller School of Medicine, Jackson Memorial Hospital, Miami, Florida

CONTRIBUTORS

DONALD E. BAXTER, MD, Department of Orthopedic Surgery, Baylor College of Medicine, Houston, Texas

TIMOTHY P. CHARLTON, MD, Assistant Professor of Orthopaedic Surgery, Keck School of Medicine, University of Southern California, Los Angeles, California

JEAN ALLAIN COLLUMBIER, MD, Clinique de l'Union, Toulouse, France

JONATHAN T. DELAND, MD, Chief, Foot and Ankle Service, Hospital for Special Surgery, New York, New York

MEGAN GOULART, BS, Medical Student, Weill Medical College of Cornell University, New York, New York

WILLIAM G. HAMILTON, MD, Orthopaedic Associates of New York; Clinical Professor of Orthopaedics, Columbia University of Physicians and Surgeons; Senior Attending, St. Lukes-Roosevelt Hospital, New York, New York

CHRISTOPHER W. HODGKINS, MD, Orthopaedic Surgery Resident, Department of Orthopaedic Surgery, University of Miami, Miller School of Medicine, Jackson Memorial Hospital, Miami, Florida

JOHN G. KENNEDY, MD, MMSc, MCh, FRCSI, FRCS (Orth), Assistant Professor of Orthopaedic Surgery, Hospital for Special Surgery, New York, New York

PADHRAIG F. O'LOUGHLIN, MD, Research Fellow, Foot and Ankle Department, Hospital for Special Surgery, New York, New York

MARTIN J. O'MALLEY, MD, Associate Professor of Medicine, Hospital for Special Surgery, New York, New York

VICTOR R. PRISK, MD, Foot and Ankle Department, Hospital for Special Surgery, New York, New York

CLINICS IN SPORTS MEDICINE

Foot and Ankle Injuries in Dance

CONTENTS
VOLUME 27 • NUMBER 2 • APRIL 2008

Foreword   **ix**
Mark D. Miller

Preface   **xi**
John G. Kennedy and Christopher W. Hodgkins

Ankle Sprains and Instability in Dancers   **247**
Padhraig F. O'Loughlin, Christopher W. Hodgkins,
and John G. Kennedy

> Ankle inversion injuries are the most common traumatic injuries in dancers. Ankle stability is integral to normal mobilization and to minimizing the risk for ankle sprain. The ability of the dynamic and static stabilizers of the ankle joint to maintain their structural integrity is a major component of the normal gait cycle. In the world of dance, this quality assumes even greater importance given the range of movement and stresses imposed on the ankle during various dance routines.

Posterior Ankle Pain in Dancers   **263**
William G. Hamilton

> Treatment of dancers can be as challenging as it is rewarding. Dancers often have unusual difficulties related to the altered kinesiology required by their individual dance form. A thorough understanding of these movements helps guide the physician to the cause of the disability, particularly in the setting of overuse injuries. This knowledge, coupled with a careful physical examination, is essential for the accurate diagnosis and treatment of the dancer, who is both artist and athlete.

Tendon Injuries in Dance   **279**
Christopher W. Hodgkins, John G. Kennedy,
and Padhraigh F. O'Loughlin

> Professional ballet dancers require an extraordinary anatomic, physiologic, and psychologic makeup to achieve and sustain their level of ability and activity. They are subject to a myriad of injuries as a result of the extreme demands of this profession. Tendon injuries are common and often coexist with other pathologies of the bone, ligaments, and psyche. It is critical that the dance doctor not examine the tendon injury in isolation, but rather the cause of the injury, either intrinsic from anatomic malalignment or from external sources, including poor form.

Posterior Tibial Tendon Tears in Dancers 289
Jonathan T. Deland and William G. Hamilton

Posterior tibial tendon tears in dancers are uncommon. No case series of such injuries has been presented. The injury does however occur, and should be differentiated from the more common causes of medial hind-foot symptoms in dancers. The relevant anatomy, biomechanics, and differential diagnosis are presented followed by a summary of four cases.

Foot and Ankle Fractures in Dancers 295
Megan Goulart, Martin J. O'Malley, Christopher W. Hodgkins, and Timothy P. Charlton

Fractures in the dance population are common. Radiography, CT, MRI, and bone scan should be used as necessary to arrive at the correct diagnosis after meticulous physical examination. Treatment should address the fracture itself and any surrounding problems such as nutritional/hormonal issues and training/performance techniques and regimens. Compliance issues in this population are a concern, so treatment strategies should be tailored accordingly. Stress fractures in particular can present difficulties to the treating physician and may require prolonged treatment periods. This article addresses stress fractures of the fibula, calcaneus, navicular, and second metatarsal; fractures of the fifth metatarsal, sesamoids, and phalanges; and dislocation of toes.

Forefoot Injuries in Dancers 305
Victor R. Prisk, Padhraig F. O'Loughlin, and John G. Kennedy

Dancers, particularly ballet dancers, are artists and athletes. In dance, the choreographer acts as a sculptor, using the dancer as a medium of expression. This often entails placing the dancer's body in positions that require extraordinary flexibility and movement, which requires controlled power and endurance. Ballet and other forms of dance can be highly demanding activities, with a lifetime injury incidence of up to 90%. Ballet is stressful particularly on the dancer's forefoot. The en pointe position of maximal plantarflexion through the forefoot, mid-foot, and hindfoot requires tremendous flexibility and strength that only can be attained safely through many years of training. The forces experienced by the toes and metatarsals are extraordinary.

Bunions in Dancers 321
John G. Kennedy and Jean Allain Collumbier

Although dancers put a great deal of stress through the first metatarso-phalangeal joint (MTPJ), it is unlikely that dancing causes bunions; however, such forces may produce an environment in which bunions may develop. It is best to employ conservative measures rather than surgical intervention in dancers who have a painful bunion. Any surgery on the first MTPJ will adversely affect dorsiflexion of this joint, which is a critical motion for dancers. Two types of bunions (slowly progressive and rapidly progressive) are commonly seen; arthritic bunions occur in dancers who have mild arthrosis and loss of cartilage on the head of the first MTPJ. Secondary problems arising from bunions include metatarsalgia, stress fractures, sesamoiditis, and flexor hallucis longus tendonitis.

Nerve Disorders in Dancers 329

John G. Kennedy and Donald E. Baxter

Dancers are required to perform at the extreme of physiologic and functional limits. Under such conditions, peripheral nerves are prone to compression. Entrapment neuropathies in dance can be related to the sciatic nerve or from a radiculopathy related to posture or a hyperlordosis. The most reproducible and reliable method of diagnosis is a careful history and clinical examination. This article reviews several nerve disorders encountered in dancers, including interdigital neuromas, tarsal tunnel syndrome, medial hallucal nerve compression, anterior tarsal tunnel syndrome, superficial and deep peroneal nerve entrapment, and sural nerve entrapment.

Index 335

CLINICS IN SPORTS MEDICINE

FORTHCOMING ISSUES

July 2008

Sports Injury Outcomes and Prevention
Joseph M. Hart, PhD, *Guest Editor*

October 2008

Shoulder Problems in Athletes
Benjamin S. Shaffer, MD, *Guest Editor*

January 2009

Future Trends in Sports Medicine
Scott A. Rodeo, MD, *Guest Editor*

RECENT ISSUES

January 2008

International Perspectives
Lyle J. Micheli, MD
Guest Editor

October 2007

ACL Graft and Fixation Choices
Jon K. Sekiya, MD, and Steven B. Cohen, MD
Guest Editors

July 2007

Infectious Disease and Sports Medicine
James R. Borchers, MD, and Thomas M. Best, MD, PhD, FACSM
Guest Editors

Clin Sports Med 27 (2008) ix

CLINICS IN SPORTS MEDICINE

Foreword

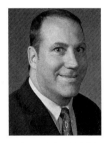

Mark D. Miller, MD

Consulting Editor

lthough some may not consider dance a sport, I would beg to differ. These athletes undergo rigorous training and routines and are subject to a variety of unique and difficult injuries. Most of these injuries involve the foot and ankle, and this issue of *Clinics in Sports Medicine* focuses on these problems. Drs. John G. Kennedy and Christopher W. Hodgkins, who are responsible for the care of a large number of these athletes, have put together an excellent treatise on the treatment of dancers. This issue covers the gambit of injuries, including tendon injuries, ankle problems, forefoot injuries, nerve disorders, and even fractures. Please enjoy this issue and, as Leo Sayer would say: "You make me feel like dancing," so dance the night away!

Mark D. Miller, MD
Department of Orthopaedic Surgery
Division of Sports Medicine
University of Virginia Health System
P.O. Box 800753
UVA Dept of Orthopaedic Surgery
Charlottesville, VA 22908-0159, USA

E-mail address: mdm3p@virginia.edu

0278-5919/08/$ – see front matter
doi:10.1016/j.csm.2008.01.004

Clin Sports Med 27 (2008) xi–xii

CLINICS IN SPORTS MEDICINE

ELSEVIER
SAUNDERS

Preface

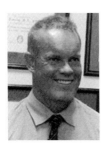
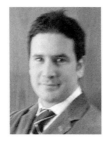

John G. Kennedy, MD, MMSc, MCh, FRCSI, FRCS (Orth), and
Christopher W. Hodgkins, MD

Guest Editors

Ballet has all the elements of the arts in its makeup: drama, poetry, literature, painting, sculpture, design, music, and, of course, dance. Dancers, both male and female, are the physical means by which the choreographer sculpts a composition of expressive motion. From an early age, the dancer must learn to be an artist, gymnast, and athlete. Most ballet dancers train for a minimum of 10 years before attaining the skill set necessary to join a corps de ballet. Very few dancers develop into soloists, and fewer still attain the role of principle ballerina. Throughout this time of training, the body is placed under great strain, and it is by a process of natural selection that those dancers who are flexible and technically proficient survive the rigors of training to advance further still. The grace and art of the ballet performance belie the great physical strain on the body as a whole—the foot and ankle in particular. This group of athletes may often confound the clinical examiner by minimizing the injury due to economic and professional pressures.

This issue provides the orthopaedist with a comprehensive look at the more common foot and ankle injuries sustained in dance, paying special attention to successfully detecting and treating these injuries in dancers. While this unique

0278-5919/08/$ – see front matter
doi:10.1016/j.csm.2008.01.003

population will always present a great challenge, careful and committed attention will produce rewarding results.

John G. Kennedy, MD, MMSc, MCh, FRCSI, FRCS (Orth)
Hospital for Special Surgery
523 East 72nd Street, Suite 514
New York, NY 10021, USA

E-mail address: kennedyj@hss.edu

Christopher W. Hodgkins, MD
Department of Orthopaedic Surgery
University of Miami, Miller School of Medicine
Jackson Memorial Hospital
Ryder Trauma Center
P.O. Box 016960 (D-27)
Miami, FL 33101, USA

E-mail address: chodgkins@med.miami.edu

Clin Sports Med 27 (2008) 247–262

CLINICS IN SPORTS MEDICINE

ELSEVIER
SAUNDERS

Ankle Sprains and Instability in Dancers

Padhraig F. O'Loughlin, MD[a],*, Christopher W. Hodgkins, MD[b],
John G. Kennedy, MD, MMSc, MCh, FRCSI, FRCS (Orth)[a]

[a]Foot and Ankle Department, Hospital for Special Surgery, 523 East 72nd Street,
Suite 514, New York, NY 10021, USA
[b]Department of Orthopaedic Surgery, University of Miami, Miller School of Medicine, Jackson
Memorial Hospital, Ryder Trauma Center, P.O. Box 016960 (D-27), Miami, FL 33101, USA

It takes an athlete to dance, but an artist to be a dancer.
—Shanna LaFleur.

Ankle inversion injuries are the most common traumatic injuries in dancers [1]. Ankle stability is integral to normal mobilization and to minimizing the risk for ankle sprain. The ability of the dynamic and static stabilizers of the ankle joint to maintain their structural integrity is a major component of the normal gait cycle. In the world of dance, this quality assumes even greater importance given the range of movement and stresses imposed on the ankle during various dance routines. Dancing is a unique combination of artistry and athleticism.

INCIDENCE

In the general population, the incidence of ankle sprain is high. Ligament injuries to the lateral ankle ligaments are shown, in several studies, to be the most common sports-related injuries, accounting for approximately 25% of all sports-related injuries [2–8]. Other studies cite their incidence as approximately 5000 injuries per day in the United Kingdom and 23,000 per day in the United States [3,4,9].

Foot and ankle injuries in dancers are common, with rates of 17% to 24% per 100 in modern dancers and 67% to 95% per 100% among professional ballet dancers [1,10–14]. The feet and ankles of dancers are particularly vulnerable to injury and represent 34% to 62% per 100 of all injuries reported [1,10–14]. This may be in part because dancers have a greater incidence of cavus feet, predisposing to lateral ankle stress. Female ballet dancers have a higher incidence of foot and ankle injuries than male, most likely due to

*Corresponding author. E-mail address: oloughlinp@hss.edu (P.F. O'Loughlin).

0278-5919/08/$ – see front matter
doi:10.1016/j.csm.2007.12.006

the amount of time spent in the pointe position [1]. In professional dancers in musical theater, foot and ankle injuries are reported as comprising 23% to 45% per 100 of all injuries [15–18].

In a study by Wiesler and colleagues [11] of 101 ballet and 47 modern dance students, 56% reported lower-limb injuries, most common being ankle sprains (28% of all dancers). The dancers were studied for a year, and during this time ankle sprain represented 13.8% of all the injuries reported, second only to tendonitis in terms of frequency. Within the dancing population, this is an issue with significant implications for performance, progression, and career. This consequently has an impact on the figures reported given that dancers often continue to dance through injury and seek treatment only when they are physically unable to perform or compete. This is an important consideration for treatment so as to prevent a cycle of recurrent injury that has a detrimental impact on a dancer's career.

ETIOLOGY AND BIOMECHANICS

Improper jump landings and rolling over the lateral aspect of the foot while on demi-pointe are typical mechanisms of injury. In these positions, the foot is loaded in plantarflexion and inversion, typically stressing the anterior talofibular ligament (ATFL).

Ankle stability is related to the bony architecture and the soft tissue constraints. The primary dynamic constraints are the peroneal tendons and flexor tendons. The primary passive constraints are the lateral ligament complex, extensor retinaculum, peroneal retinaculum, talocalcaneal ligaments, and interosseous ligaments.

Biomechanics should be an integral consideration when assessing dancers, as malalignment elsewhere in the body could contribute to susceptibility to ankle sprain. Thus, an ankle injury should not be looked at as a single entity but as a component of the greater biokinetic chain.

Kinetic chain dysfunctions are common in ballet dancers, in particular with overuse injuries, which commonly follow ankle sprains. They may represent a secondary phenomenon that developed in response to the compensatory movement changes caused by the initial injury. This may be more likely if dancers continue to train and perform despite injury. These dysfunctions, however, may have been long-standing and a causative factor in the injury.

Accordingly, it is essential to examine the entire chain thoroughly for functional movements when dealing with an injury, because identification and treatment of kinetic chain dysfunction is important in the rehabilitation of dancing athletes and in prevention of reinjury or chronic damage.

ANKLE INSTABILITY

Risk Factors

In recurrent ankle sprains of the ankle or chronic ankle instability, there are certain factors that most be considered to plan appropriate management. Those general considerations that affect athletes and their propensity to ankle sprain apply as readily to dancers. Anatomic malalignment, inadequate conditioning, and improper technique all are important factors.

Dance-Specific Risk Factors

Environmental issues, such as dancing surface, ambient temperature, and size of the performance are important considerations [1]. Frequency and duration of performance, with a consequent increase in training or rehearsal time, also have an impact on frequency of injury [19].

Inversion ankle sprains are most common when dancers lose balance while landing from a jump with an ankle in plantarflexion [19]. The specific ligament that is injured depends on the position of the ankle at the time of landing.

Dancing en pointe

Female ballet dancers frequently adopt the full-pointe position, which requires marked plantarflexion with the toes in a neutral position relative to the longitudinal axis of the foot (Fig. 1). In full pointe, the ankle is relatively stable, as the posterior lip of the tibia rests and locks on the calcaneus, and the subtalar joint is locked with the heel and forefoot in varus. Thus, a midfoot sprain is more likely in this position than an ankle sprain [19]. With slight dorsiflexion, however, this complex releases, placing greater pressure on the lateral ligament complex and rendering the ankle more vulnerable to an inversion injury. As the ankle inverts progressively, the strain on the other ankle ligament increases. In plantarflexion, the ATFL assumes a vertical position while the narrow portion of the talus is in position within the ankle mortise. In this position, there

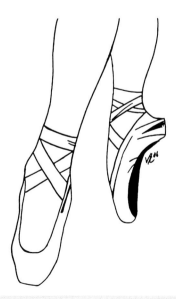

Fig. 1. En pointe.

is minimal support offered by the calcaneofibular ligament (CFL) and syndesmotic ligaments. Demi-pointe is a variation of this position (Figs. 2 and 3).

Turnout

In ballet, turnout is an external rotation of the leg, causing the knee and foot to turn outward, away from the center of the body. This rotation allows for greater extension of the leg, especially when raising it to the side and rear. Turnout is deemed essential to classical ballet technique and is the basis on which all ballet movement follows. Thus, ballet dancers are encouraged to develop this posture.

It may cause stress, however, on dancers' lower back, hip, and lower extremities and put them at risk for injury, including ankle injury. Coplan [20] established that, based on self-reported history of low back and lower extremity injuries, ballet dancers have a greater risk for injury if they reach a turnout position that is greater than their available bilateral passive hip external rotation range of motion. Alternatively, Negus and colleagues [21] found, in a study of 29 ballet dancers, that 93.1% reported a history of nontraumatic injuries and 41.4% a history of traumatic injuries. Number and severity of nontraumatic injuries were associated with a reduced functional turnout but not with the range of external rotation at the hip. This study was based on the theory that overuse or nontraumatic dance injuries often are attributed to faults in technique, with poor turnout and inappropriate compensatory strategies major factors. In summary, it is evident that turnout has an important role in dancers' injuries, including insults to the ankle joint.

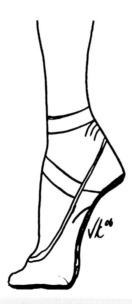

Fig. 2. En demi-pointe.

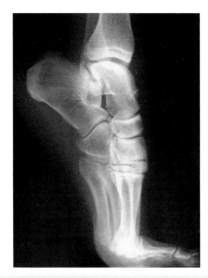

Fig. 3. Radiograph of dancer en demi-pointe.

Footwear

There is a specific pointe shoe that acts a major additional stabilizer of the foot en pointe. This is demonstrated in a cadaveric study [22]. The pointe shoes traditionally have been constructed with layers of paper, glue, and materials, such as satin, canvas, or leather. This design has not changed dramatically over the years. Although the shoes are hard to begin with, they are broken in quickly and become soft and pliable. A principal dancer may use two to three pairs of these shoes per performance [1]. These softened shoes with compromised supportive properties themselves may contribute to ankle injury.

Thus, dancers' foot wear should be examined and fitting of dance shoes, especially pointe shoes, should be performed only by an expert who is suitably trained and who understands the nature and proper fit of the shoes.

LATERAL ANKLE INJURY

Lateral Ligament Complex

This is comprised of three major ligaments: the ATFL, CFL, and posterior talofibular ligament (PTFL). As with other athletes, in dancers, it is the ATFL that is injured most frequently.

Anterior talofibular ligament

The ATFL is an intra-articular thickening of the anterolateral portion of the joint capsule, which is on average 10 mm in length, 8 mm in width, and 2 mm in thickness. It is the weakest of the ankle ligaments and, given its orientation, the most commonly injured of the ligaments of the lateral ligament complex.

The ATFL is the primary restraint to plantarflexion and inversion. When the foot is in the neutral position, it essentially is parallel to the axis of the foot, whereas when the foot is maximally plantarflexed, it becomes parallel to the axis of the lower limb. Biomechanically, this ligament limits internal rotation within the mortice of the ankle joint and limits adduction in plantarflexion.

Given the frequency with which dancers and, in particular, ballet dancers are called on to plantarflex (eg, demi-pointe and pointe), there is an increased risk for an inversion injury. This risk is increased if a dancer has sustained previous sprains without appropriate treatment and rehabilitation.

Calcaneofibular ligament

The CFL is extracapular, cordlike, and stronger than the ATFL. It acts as the floor of the peroneal sheath and thus is associated with tears of the sheath and tendon itself. It spans the ankle and subtalar joint with its origin below the ATFL and not at the distal tip of the fibula. Biomechanically the CFL is the main lateral ankle stabilizer in neutral.

Posterior talofibular ligament

The PTFL is the strongest of the three primary lateral stabilizers and aligned horizontally when the foot is in the neutral position. It rarely is injured. Biomechanically, it restricts external rotation in dorsiflexion.

Grading of Lateral Ankle Sprains

A grading system for ankle sprains was described by Kannus and Renstrom [4], which divided the injuries into mild (ligamentous strain or stretch), moderate (partial tear), and severe (complete tear). de Bie and colleagues [23], however, have argued that this grading system should be considered as purely theoretic because it has no therapeutic or prognostic consequences. In practice, however, the grading system can provide a guideline for treatment once specific patients being treated, their activities, and their expectations are considered. This is extremely important for dancers.

Presentations and Assessment

Dancers complain of swelling and lateral ankle pain. If dancers are unable to bear weight, a fracture may be present. Any bony tenderness over an ankle or lateral foot should alert an examiner that radiographs are required. If symptoms do not improve in a week, then a CT scan of the ankle and midfoot should be obtained to identify osteochondral fractures of the talus or occult fractures of the tarsal bones.

The grade of injury can be investigated subjectively by virtue of a complete history and objectively by physical examination (eg, anterior drawer test, talar tilt test, and radiography). Klenerman and van Dijk and colleagues advocate delaying a physical examination for 4 to 7 days post injury to allow for a more accurate diagnosis while excluding a fracture [24–26].

The Ottawa ankle rules [27–29] represent an algorithm that aims to prevent unnecessary x-ray investigations in the setting of acute ankle sprains. They recommend ankle radiographs if patients are not capable of taking three steps (limping is permitted) after an injury or if there is tenderness over the midportion or crest of the medial or lateral malleoluls from the tip to 6 cm proximally. Young dancers who have open physes may require radiographs more frequently. Radiographic findings include fractures, widening of the ankle mortise, avulsion fragments from the malleoli, and osteochondral injuries to the talar dome or tibial plafond. Attention also should be paid to the lateral process of the talus, the os trigonum, the anterior process of the calcaneus, and the proximal portion of the fifth metatarsal. In dancers, the os is at particular risk and an MRI often is helpful in delineating an os trigonum from a fractured os or Stieda lesion, which can present with lateral ankle pain.

MEDIAL ANKLE INJURY

Although posterior tibial tendon pathology is common in other athletes, it is rare in dancers for many reasons. Typically, a dancer's foot is cavus, which tends to protect him or her from tibialis posterior pathology as opposed to a more planus foot. Also, when a dancer is in equinus, the posterior tibial tendon is relatively shortened as the subtalar joint is inverted.

Although these medial injuries occur infrequently in dancers, they typically are associated with a pronated foot landing off balance. If a foot is in plantar-flexion, the anterior deltoid ligament is maximally affected, with the tension greatest in the deltoid in this position. Similarly, when a foot is flat on the ground and hyperpronated, a tear occurs in the midportion of the deltoid.

An accessory bone, the os subtibiale, can be found in the substance of the deltoid ligament. When injured, it may manifest as a trigger point of pain when ligamentous healing should be complete. A local injection of a steroid can be successful in treating this complaint.

Chronic strain of the deltoid ligament from poor form in the rolling in (pronation) of the foot is a common overuse injury in dancers. Chronic strain of the anterior aspect of the deltoid ligament, anchored to the capsule of the talonavicular joint, may predispose an ankle to chronic rotatory instability.

Recalcitrant medial ankle pain may be caused by an osteochondral lesion of the talus after a sprain (Fig. 4). Clinical suspicion warrants further investigation with CT or MRI to demonstrate the extent of the lesion. The size of the osteochondral lesion determines the most appropriate treatment. Microfracture treatment, chondrocyte transplant, allograft implants, and osteochondral grafting are available techniques.

Osteochondral autologous transplant surgery is indicated for large lesions (typically greater than 8 mm) with cartilage collapse or deficit and extensive underlying bone necrosis. The lesion is cored out of the talus and filled with osteochondral autograft, commonly from a non–weight-bearing location in the lateral femoral condyle (Fig. 5).

ASSOCIATED INJURIES

Inversion injury (Table 1) can cause tearing of the syndesmosis, diastasis of the distal tibiofibular joint, and a fracture of the proximal fibula (a Maisonneuve

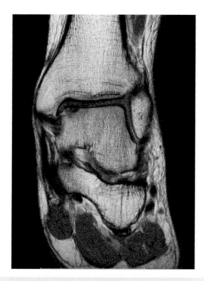

Fig. 4. Osteochondral lesion of medial talar dome.

fracture). Examination reveals significant tenderness and swelling over the proximal fibula and a positive squeeze test. Standard ankle radiographs may show widening of the mortise but does not reveal the fracture. If clinically indicated, full-length leg radiographs should be performed.

Longitudinal tears or subluxation of the peroneal tendons can cause persistent lateral pain, swelling, clicking, and a sense of something moving out of

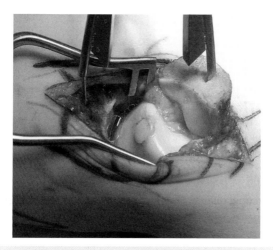

Fig. 5. Intraoperative image of osteochondral defect successfully cored out and filled with cylindric autologous bone graft from ipsilateral knee.

Table 1
Associated injuries and the differential diagnosis of residual pain/discomfort in dancer post sprain

Bone	Soft tissue
Avulsion fracture of distal fibula	Avulsion of extensor digitorum brevis
Accessory ossicle or os subfibulare	Soft tissue entrapment
Os calcis fracture	Sinus tarsi syndrome
Os perineum fracture	Syndesmotic disruption
Later process of talus fracture	Anterolateral gutter scarring or Ferkel's phenomenon
Cuboid subluxation	Talar irritation from a slip of the ATFL inserting at the extreme tip of the fibula or the Bassett's ligament
Os trigonum fracture (Sheperd's fracture)	Peroneal tendon dislocation or subluxation
Proximal fibula fracture (Maisonneuve injury)	Impingement of a lateral branch of the deep peroneal nerve

place. Resisted eversion with an examiner's fingers over the posterior aspect of the lateral malleolus can provoke and demonstrate tendon subluxation. MRI can demonstrate intrasubstance rupture or persistent tendinopathy. These injuries frequently require surgical repair.

Subluxation of the cuboid is common in dancers and may occur in association with inversion ankle sprains or with repetitive plantar dorsiflexion as a dancer goes up and down en pointe [30]. The medial border of the cuboid generally subluxates in a plantar direction, resulting in dorsal displacement of the fourth metatarsal base and plantar displacement of the fourth metatarsal head. Cuboid dysfunction interferes with the function of the peroneal tendons and always should be a prime consideration in dancers who have peroneal tendonitis.

Patients who have cuboid subluxation present with persistent lateral midfoot pain, often after a sprain that does not respond to usual treatments. Dancers may be unable to bear weight or walk normally and frequently have difficulty rolling through the foot onto pointe. Physical findings include significant tenderness over the cuboid bone, reduced mobility of the cuboid compared with the opposite foot, reduced lateral midfoot mobility on passive pronation and supination, a step-off at the base of the fourth metatarsal, and a plantar-flexed fourth metatarsal head. Treatment is directed at mobilizing the rear- and midfoot, adducting the forefoot, and then reducing the cuboid using a squeeze technique as described by Marshall and Hamilton [30].

Another differential diagnosis for residual foot pain after ankle sprain is that of nerve impingement. Typically, nerve impingement is attributed to compression of the deep peroneal nerve by the inferior extensor retinaculum and surrounding structures described as anterior tarsal tunnel syndrome. This syndrome is rare, yet the symptoms from this nerve compression have been accepted universally as dysesthesia in the first web space associated with medial foot pain.

The lateral branch of the deep peroneal nerve can cause symptoms that are distinct from typical presentations for foot and ankle maladies [31]. Patients generally report anterolateral foot pain with radiation to the lateral tarsometatarsal joints. This usually is caused by compression of the lateral branch of the deep peroneal nerve at two distinct points: the superior border of the extensor digitorum brevis and over the anterolateral aspect of the talar head. The condition can be diagnosed by careful clinical examination, including a maneuver in which the foot is inverted and plantarflexed. In this position, the lateral branch of the deep peroneal nerve is stretched over the head of the talus and can often be palpated. The two points of nerve compression are emphasized in this provocative position, facilitating reproducible nerve compression testing. To confirm diagnosis, a small amount of local anesthetic agent can be infiltrated at approximately the point of compression. Kennedy and colleagues [31] advocate surgical release in patients whose symptoms return after an initial resolution after local anesthetic block.

MANAGEMENT
Treatment of Lateral Ligament Complex Injuries With Respect to Grade
Grade I
Grade I typically is a sprain or stretch of the ATFL and typically a stable injury, requiring rest, ice, compression, and elevation for 48 hours. Thereafter, motion is encouraged with a light compressive bandage. Dancers can begin light workouts at 48 hours, with the aid of a brace or Aircast splint. Initially, therapy should concentrate on range of motion. After 4 or 5 days, dancers begin to wean out of the brace and initiate proprioception, balance, and peroneal strengthening exercises.

Grade II
Partial tear of the ATFL occasionally may involve damage to the CFL also. A positive drawer sign but negative talar tilt frequently is observed. Treatment begins with immobilization in a cam walker or Aircast splint for up to 6 weeks. Initially, physical therapy should focus on regaining appropriate range of motion. Thereafter, a triple-phase rehabilitation program, including peroneal strengthening, balance retraining, and proprioceptive conditioning should be initiated early.

Grade III
This grade of injury is typically unstable. The ATFL and the CFL commonly are injured. In addition, the drawer sign and talar tilt are positive. Treatment traditionally is immobilization for up to 6 weeks. In professional dancers, primary repair can be an option, and the Brostrom-Gould usually can be performed 1 week after the injury with predictable results and return of function [32]. Regardless of the treatment used, attention must be paid to re-establishing a functionally stable joint and to restoration of the baseline range of motion. This is crucial in dancers to maximize the chances of returning to the previous level of performance and ability.

A comprehensive literature evaluation and meta-analysis showed that early functional treatment by comparison to anatomic reconstruction produced the fastest recovery of ankle mobility and earliest return to activity without affecting mechanical stability [33].

Closed-chain balance and proprioception activities, along with peroneal muscle strengthening, improves neuromuscular control of the ankle. Therapists must be familiar with the modalities needed to achieve these goals to optimize outcomes in these dancers.

Studies have evaluated proprioception in dancers [34,35]. Female dancers showed no difference compared with nondancers in proprioception ability. Dancers who had sustained an ankle sprain had altered sensorimotor control compared with those who did not have prior injury, despite having returned to full-time performing and completing proprioception training.

Conservative Versus Surgical Treatment of Ankle Sprains and Instability in Dancers

Currently, there is no conclusive answer to this treatment dilemma regarding dancers, athletes, or the general population. A Cochrane meta-analysis of 2562 patients comparing surgery to conservative treatment in the setting of an acute ankle sprain failed to demonstrate a clearly superior treatment approach [33]. There was some evidence to suggest that surgery may provide benefit over conservative treatment in some less important secondary outcomes, but the heterogeneity in results for primary outcomes means the evidence presented must be interpreted with caution. The conclusions were that treatment should be made on an individual basis, carefully weighing the relative benefits and risks for each option. Given the risk for surgical complications and higher costs, the best option for most patients was deemed a conservative approach to acute ankle sprains with close follow-up to identify those who remained symptomatic.

This approach rings true for dancers. The choice of treatment for dancers should be tailored specifically to the specific injury and risk factors. A close follow-up is important so as not to miss any subtle associated injuries that might have a negative impact on performance, leave dancers vulnerable to reinjury, or precipitate a more severe or chronic condition.

CHRONIC ANKLE INSTABILITY

de Vries and colleagues [36] define chronic ankle sprain as an injury that precipitates symptoms for more than 6 months and they believe that surgical reconstruction at this point at least should be considered. With acute ankle sprain recurrence rates as high as 70% in patients who have lateral ligament injury, it is easy to imagine how a chronic condition could evolve [37]. Yeung and colleagues [38] have established that up to 40% of initial injuries have post-sprain dysfunction.

Given the busy schedule of professional dancers, the chance of repeat injury after an initial insult to the lateral ligament complex is high. Mechanical instability and functional instability are two of the principal contributors to chronic instability [39–42].

Types of Chronic Ankle Instability

Functional instability

In functional instability, a dancer's joint motion is within normal range. Although the mechanical stabilizers of the ankle are intact, the stability or steadiness of the joint is beyond voluntary control. Simple examination techniques, such as having a dancer stand on one leg, can precipitate momentary oscillation before eventually achieving a stable balance.

Matsusaka and colleagues [43] have attributed functional instability to disturbed proprioception and advocated physical therapy with specific focus on co-ordination and strength while re-establishing proprioception and thus stability. Baier and Hopf [44] described the benefit of taping and braces via direct mechanical support and suggested an additional positive effect by enhancement of proprioception through skin pressure. Boyle and Negus [45] studied the joint position awareness in an ankle that sustained recurrent sprains and noted significant differences in terms of proprioception compared with an uninjured joint.

Mechanical instability

With the mechanical form of ankle instability, there is compromise of the normal anchors of the ankle joint such that the normal limits of joint motion are exceeded. This readily is evident on performing an anterior drawer or talar tilt test.

Combined functional and mechanical instability

Although mechanical and functional instability may occur in isolation, studies demonstrate that it most likely is a combination of the two conditions that contributes to chronic instability [40,41,46]. Other studies discuss this same topic, proposing that chronic ankle instability with increased ligament laxity is accompanied by a proprioceptive deficit [47–49].

By contrast, the absence of one form of instability may compensate for the presence of the other. This is supported by abnormal laxity not always resulting in symptomatic instability.

Treatment of Chronic Instability

The majority of people make a full recovery when treated conservatively but a cohort may need to progress to surgery [50]. Up to 20% of patients may continue to suffer from lateral ankle instability after acute injury despite adequate physical therapy [51].

Surgical options

Surgery to address ankle instability that results from severe lateral ligament injury commonly is divided into those procedures that aim to restore the previous anatomy and those that create checkreins.

Those that seek to restore correct anatomy involve direct ligament repair and include the Brostrom and modified Brostrom procedures [8,32]. The checkrein procedures involve tendon transfers and include the Elmslie (fascia lata) [52], Watson-Jones (peroneus brevis) [53,54], Evans (peroneus brevis) [55], Chrisman-Snook [56], and Larsen (peroneus brevis) procedures [57].

Hamilton and colleagues [32] have described the efficacy of the modified Brostrom technique in restoring function and stability in dancers. In addition, retrospective comparative studies have suggested that anatomic restoration shows superior results in the long term [58,59]. Hennrikus and colleagues [46] have shown a significantly higher rate of nerve damage in the Chrisman-Snook procedure.

Specific treatment considerations with respect to dancers

Early and aggressive treatment of ankle sprains is essential in dancers. Dancing en pointe necessitates maximal mobility of all joints of the lower leg, ankle, and foot, with restricted motion leading to difficulty with technique, further injury, and, ultimately, implications for a dancer's career.

Swelling contributes to loss of motion and should be minimized. Simple techniques may be used, such as use of icing and compression taping with horseshoe pads. The subtalar joint and the talocalcaneal ligament frequently are injured in inversion sprains. Subtalar sprains are linked to chronic giving way and limitations of ankle motion [60], which can result in significant disability for dancers. Range-of-motion exercises, therefore, are initiated as early as possible to maintain and restore mobility of the ankle and subtalar joints.

Strength training with specific emphasis on the everters should be performed in the neutral position and, crucially, with the foot in the plantarflexed, pointe position. Flexibility of the gastrocnemius and soleus muscles is critical. Functional mobility drills should be used first at the barre and subsequently on the center of the dance floor before returning to full dance.

SUMMARY

Aggressive treatment of the sprained ankle is essential to maintaining foot and ankle mobility and preventing prolonged disability and subsequent overuse injuries.

References

[1] Kadel NJ. Foot and ankle injuries in dance. Phys Med Rehabil Clin N Am 2006;17: 813–26, vii.

[2] Balduini FC, Vegso JJ, Torg JS, et al. Management and rehabilitation of ligamentous injuries to the ankle. Sports Med 1987;4:364–80.

[3] Karlsson J, Sancone M. Management of acute ligament injuries of the ankle. Foot Ankle Clin 2006;11:521–30.

[4] Kannus P, Renstrom P. Treatment for acute tears of the lateral ligaments of the ankle. Operation, cast, or early controlled mobilization. J Bone Joint Surg Am 1991;73:305–12.

[5] Brostrom L. Sprained ankles. 3. Clinical observations in recent ligament ruptures. Acta Chir Scand 1965;130:560–9.

[6] Brostrom L, Sundelin P. Sprained ankles. IV. Histologic changes in recent and "chronic" ligament ruptures. Acta Chir Scand 1966;132:248–53.

[7] Brostrom L. Sprained ankles. V. Treatment and prognosis in recent ligament ruptures. Acta Chir Scand 1966;132:537–50.

[8] Brostrom L. Sprained ankles. VI. Surgical treatment of "chronic" ligament ruptures. Acta Chir Scand 1966;132:551–65.

[9] Lynch SA, Renstrom PA. Treatment of acute lateral ankle ligament rupture in the athlete. Conservative versus surgical treatment. Sports Med 1999;27:61–71.

[10] Nilsson C, Leanderson J, Wykman A, et al. The injury panorama in a Swedish professional ballet company. Knee Surg Sports Traumatol Arthrosc 2001;9:242–6.

[11] Wiesler ER, Hunter DM, Martin DF, et al. Ankle flexibility and injury patterns in dancers. Am J Sports Med 1996;24:754–7.

[12] Garrick JG, Requa RK. Ballet injuries. An analysis of epidemiology and financial outcome. Am J Sports Med 1993;21:586–90.

[13] Byhring S, Bo K. Musculoskeletal injuries in the Norwegian National Ballet: a prospective cohort study. Scand J Med Sci Sports 2002;12:365–70.

[14] Bronner S, Ojofeitimi S, Rose D. Injuries in a modern dance company: effect of comprehensive management on injury incidence and time loss. Am J Sports Med 2003;31:365–73.

[15] Washington EL. Musculoskeletal injuries in theatrical dancers: site frequency, and severity. Am J Sports Med 1978;6:75–98.

[16] Rovere GD, Webb LX, Gristina AG, et al. Musculoskeletal injuries in theatrical dance students. Am J Sports Med 1983;11:195–8.

[17] Evans RW, Evans RI, Carvajal S. Survey of injuries among West End performers. Occup Environ Med 1998;55:585–93.

[18] Evans RW, Evans RI, Carvajal S, et al. A survey of injuries among Broadway performers. Am J Public Health 1996;86:77–80.

[19] Macintyre J, Joy E. Foot and ankle injuries in dance. Clin Sports Med 2000;19:351–68.

[20] Coplan JA. Ballet dancer's turnout and its relationship to self-reported injury. J Orthop Sports Phys Ther 2002;32:579–84.

[21] Negus V, Hopper D, Briffa NK. Associations between turnout and lower extremity injuries in classical ballet dancers. J Orthop Sports Phys Ther 2005;35:307–18.

[22] Kadel N, Boenisch M, Teitz C, et al. Stability of Lisfranc joints in ballet pointe position. Foot Ankle Int 2005;26:394–400.

[23] de Bie RA, de Vet HC, van den Wildenberg FA, et al. The prognosis of ankle sprains. Int J Sports Med 1997;18:285–9.

[24] Klenerman L. The management of sprained ankle. J Bone Joint Surg Br 1998;80:11–2.

[25] van Dijk CN, Lim LS, Bossuyt PM, et al. Physical examination is sufficient for the diagnosis of sprained ankles. J Bone Joint Surg Br 1996;78:958–62.

[26] van Dijk CN, Mol BW, Lim LS, et al. Diagnosis of ligament rupture of the ankle joint. Physical examination, arthrography, stress radiography and sonography compared in 160 patients after inversion trauma. Acta Orthop Scand 1996;67:566–70.

[27] Pigman EC, Klug RK, Sanford S, et al. Evaluation of the Ottawa clinical decision rules for the use of radiography in acute ankle and midfoot injuries in the emergency department: an independent site assessment. Ann Emerg Med 1994;24:41–5.

[28] Stiell IG, Greenberg GH, McKnight RD, et al. Decision rules for the use of radiography in acute ankle injuries. Refinement and prospective validation. JAMA 1993;269:1127–32.

[29] Stiell IG, McKnight RD, Greenberg GH, et al. Implementation of the Ottawa ankle rules. JAMA 1994;271:827–32.

[30] Marshall P, Hamilton WG. Cuboid subluxation in ballet dancers. Am J Sports Med 1992;20:169–75.

[31] Kennedy JG, Brunner JB, Bohne WH, et al. Clinical importance of the lateral branch of the deep peroneal nerve. Clin Orthop Relat Res 2007;459:222–8.

[32] Hamilton WG, Thompson FM, Snow SW. The modified Brostrom procedure for lateral ankle instability. Foot Ankle 1993;14:1–7.

[33] Kerkhoffs GM, Handoll HH, de Bie R, et al. Surgical versus conservative treatment for acute injuries of the lateral ligament complex of the ankle in adults. Cochrane Database Syst Rev 2007;(2):CD000380.

[34] Leanderson J, Eriksson E, Nilsson C, et al. Proprioception in classical ballet dancers. A prospective study of the influence of an ankle sprain on proprioception in the ankle joint. Am J Sports Med 1996;24:370–4.

[35] Schmitt H, Kuni B, Sabo D. Influence of professional dance training on peak torque and proprioception at the ankle. Clin J Sport Med 2005;15:331–9.

[36] de Vries JS, Krips R, Sierevelt IN, et al. Interventions for treating chronic ankle instability. Cochrane Database Syst Rev 2006;(4):CD004124.

[37] McKay GD, Goldie PA, Payne WR, et al. Ankle injuries in basketball: injury rate and risk factors. Br J Sports Med 2001;35:103–8.

[38] Yeung MS, Chan KM, So CH, et al. An epidemiological survey on ankle sprain. Br J Sports Med 1994;28:112–6.

[39] Freeman MA. Instability of the foot after injuries to the lateral ligament of the ankle. J Bone Joint Surg Br 1965;47:669–77.

[40] Hertel J. Functional anatomy, pathomechanics, and pathophysiology of lateral ankle instability. J Athl Train 2002;37:364–75.

[41] Tropp H, Odenrick P, Gillquist J. Stabilometry recordings in functional and mechanical instability of the ankle joint. Int J Sports Med 1985;6:180–2.

[42] Hubbard TJ, Kramer LC, Denegar CR, et al. Contributing factors to chronic ankle instability. Foot Ankle Int 2007;28:343–54.

[43] Matsusaka N, Yokoyama S, Tsurusaki T, et al. Effect of ankle disk training combined with tactile stimulation to the leg and foot on functional instability of the ankle. Am J Sports Med 2001;29:25–30.

[44] Baier M, Hopf T. Ankle orthoses effect on single-limb standing balance in athletes with functional ankle instability. Arch Phys Med Rehabil 1998;79:939–44.

[45] Boyle J, Negus V. Joint position sense in the recurrently sprained ankle. Aust J Physiother 1998;44:159–63.

[46] Hennrikus WL, Mapes RC, Lyons PM, et al. Outcomes of the Chrisman-Snook and modified-Brostrom procedures for chronic lateral ankle instability. A prospective, randomized comparison. Am J Sports Med 1996;24:400–4.

[47] Halasi T, Kynsburg A, Tallay A, et al. Changes in joint position sense after surgically treated chronic lateral ankle instability. Br J Sports Med 2005;39:818–24.

[48] Larsen E. Static or dynamic repair of chronic lateral ankle instability. A prospective randomized study. Clin Orthop Relat Res 1990;257:184–92.

[49] Rosenbaum D, Engelhardt M, Becker HP, et al. Clinical and functional outcome after anatomic and nonanatomic ankle ligament reconstruction: Evans tenodesis versus periosteal flap. Foot Ankle Int 1999;20:636–9.

[50] Kerkhoffs GM, Handoll HH, de Bie R, et al. Surgical versus conservative treatment for acute injuries of the lateral ligament complex of the ankle in adults. Cochrane Database Syst Rev 2002;(3):CD000380.

[51] Karlsson J, Eriksson BI, Sward L. Early functional treatment for acute ligament injuries of the ankle joint. Scand J Med Sci Sports 1996;6:341–5.

[52] Elmslie RC. Recurrent subluxation of the ankle-joint. Ann Surg 1934;100:364–7.

[53] Gillespie HS, Boucher P. Watson-Jones repair of lateral instability of the ankle. J Bone Joint Surg Am 1971;53:920–4.

[54] Brattstrom H. Tenodesis employing the method of Watson-Jones for the treatment of recurrent subluxation of the ankle. Acta Orthop Scand 1953;23:132–6.

[55] Evans DL. Recurrent instability of the ankle; a method of surgical treatment. Proc R Soc Med 1953;46:343–4.

[56] Chrisman OD, Snook GA. Reconstruction of lateral ligament tears of the ankle. An experimental study and clinical evaluation of seven patients treated by a new modification of the Elmslie procedure. J Bone Joint Surg Am 1969;51:904–12.

[57] Larsen E. Tendon transfer for lateral ankle and subtalar joint instability. Acta Orthop Scand 1988;59:168–72.

[58] Krips R, Brandsson S, Swensson C, et al. Anatomical reconstruction and Evans tenodesis of the lateral ligaments of the ankle. Clinical and radiological findings after follow-up for 15 to 30 years. J Bone Joint Surg Br 2002;84:232–6.

[59] Krips R, van Dijk CN, Halasi T, et al. Anatomical reconstruction versus tenodesis for the treatment of chronic anterolateral instability of the ankle joint: a 2- to 10-year follow-up, multicenter study. Knee Surg Sports Traumatol Arthrosc 2000;8:173–9.

[60] Tochigi Y, Yoshinaga K, Wada Y, et al. Acute inversion injury of the ankle: magnetic resonance imaging and clinical outcomes. Foot Ankle Int 1998;19:730–4.

Clin Sports Med 27 (2008) 263–277

CLINICS IN SPORTS MEDICINE

Posterior Ankle Pain in Dancers

William G. Hamilton, MD

Orthopaedic Associates of New York, 343 West 58th Street, New York, NY 10019, USA

P osterior ankle pain is common in athletes, such as dancers, gymnasts, soccer players, and skaters, who must work or kick in the equinus position (full plantar flexion) [1–10]. A review of posterior ankle anatomy helps to explain the two common pain syndromes found in this area [11,12]. The posterior aspect of the talus has two tubercles: the medial and the lateral (Fig. 1). The lateral tubercle is the origin of the posterior talofibular ligament. The tubercle can be large or small. When it is large it is referred to as the "posterior process of the talus" or "Stieda's process." In 7% to 11% of people, this posterior process is separate from the talus and connected by a fibrous synostosis; it is then called the "os trigonum" (OT) [11,12]. The OT is the second most common accessory bone in the foot, the accessory navicular being the most common [13]. Bony impingement can occur posterolaterally when the trigonal process or OT is compressed between the posterior lip of the tibia and superior portion of the os calcis in extreme plantar flexion (Fig. 2) [9,10,14–16].

The flexor hallucis longus (FHL) tendon passes through a fibro-osseous tunnel between the two posterior tubercles as it runs from its origin on the fibula (laterally) to its insertion in the distal phalanx of the hallux (medially) (see Fig. 1). Chronic tendinitis and dysfunction within this tunnel can produce posterior medial pain (dancer's tendinitis) [1,2,5,7,17]. There are three sources of posterior ankle pain: (1) lateral (trigonal impingement); (2) medial (FHL tendinitis); and (3) a combination of both. It is important to know which syndrome one is dealing with in planning the surgical approach. If the problem is posterior impingement only, the approach is lateral. If the problem is FHL tendonitis or a combination of FHL tendonitis and posterior impingement, a medial approach should be used so that the neurovascular bundle can be adequately protected [18–21].

POSTEROMEDIAL ANKLE PAIN

Tendinitis of the FHL tendon behind the medial malleolus of the ankle is so common in dancers that it is known as "dancer's tendinitis" [2,4,7,17]. The FHL tendon is the Achilles tendon of the foot for the dancer, especially the

E-mail address: maryvelazco@covad.net

0278-5919/08/$ – see front matter
doi:10.1016/j.csm.2007.12.002

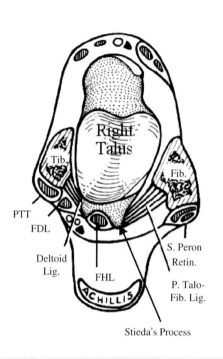

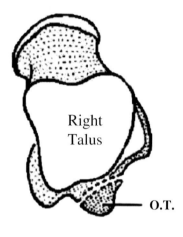

O.T. The ununited lateral
process of talus
Occurrence - 8%
Bilateral - 50%

Right
Talus

O.T.

Tib.

Fib.

PTT

FDL

Deltoid
Lig.

FHL

S. Peron
Retin.

P. Talo-
Fib. Lig.

Stieda's Process

Fig. 1. Anatomy of the posterior ankle. (*Courtesy of* W.G. Hamilton, MD, New York, NY.)

ballet dancer who works on full pointe in the toeshoe. It passes through a fibro-osseous tunnel behind the talus like a rope through a pulley. As it passes through this pulley, it is often strained. When this occurs, rather than moving smoothly in the pulley, it binds. This binding causes irritation and swelling, which causes further binding, irritation, and swelling, setting up a chronic cycle: because it is swollen and irritated, it binds; and because it binds, it is swollen and irritated. If a nodule or partial tear is present, triggering of the big toe may occur (hallux saltans) (Fig. 3). In the extreme, the tendon may become completely frozen in the sheath, causing pseudo hallux rigidus, although this is rare. This tendinitis typically responds to the usual conservative measures. Relative rest in a removable walker boot to immobilize the first Metatarsophalangeal (MP) joint is an important component of the therapy so that the chronic cycle previously described can be broken. Nonsteroidal anti-inflammatory drugs can help, but they should be used only as part of an overall treatment program and not as simply to kill the pain so that the dancer can continue dancing and ignore the symptoms. As with other tendon problems, steroid injections should be avoided in the office setting because of the danger of injecting the steroid directly into the tendon. Diagnostic and therapeutic injections can be performed into the FHL tendon sheath accurately and safely,

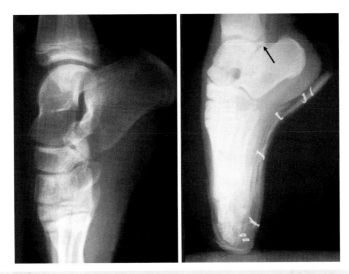

Fig. 2. Ankles without (*left*) and with (*right*) an os trigonum (*arrow*). Note difference in plantar flexion of the talus.

however, under sonographic control [22]. Failure of conservative therapy or recurrence of symptoms may be a sign of rents or longitudinal tears in the tendon [23,24]. MRI studies are not always accurate in diagnosing these partial tears. In some cases, sonography has been more accurate in evaluating the tendon than MRI studies. An indirect sign of chronic FHL tendonitis on an MRI is

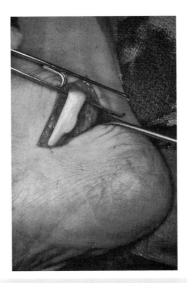

Fig. 3. Hallux saltans; a nodule on FHL tendon causing triggering of hallux.

the appearance of cysts behind the ankle (the Baker's cyst of the ankle) (Fig. 4). These usually come, not from the ankle joint, but from the chronic irritation in the FHL sheath. Ruptures of the tendon have been reported [25,26] but they are rare. On some occasions, in professional or high-level amateur dancers and athletes, FHL tendinitis may be recurrent and disabling. In refractory cases, operative tenolysis may be indicated, but only after failure of conservative treatment. The situation is similar to de Quervain's stenosing tenosynovitis in the wrist.

Thomasen [15] described a condition that bears his name: Thomasen's sign. This occurs when the muscle fibers on the FHL insert distally on the tendon and are pulled down into the tunnel when both the ankle and great toe are dorsiflexed at the same time (as in the grand plié in fifth position Fig. 5). This produces a "functional hallux rigidus" (ie, the great toe has normal motion when the ankle is plantar flexed, but does not dorsiflex when the ankle is dorsiflexed) (Fig. 6). Thomasen's sign is more of an anatomic curiosity than a pathologic condition. Many world class ballerinas have a positive Thomasen's sign in their foot and are asymptomatic. FHL tendinitis usually occurs behind the medial malleolus, but occasionally it can be found at the knot of Henry under the base of the first metatarsal where the flexor digitorum longus crosses over the FHL (jogger's foot) [27] and rarely under the head of the first metatarsal where it passes between the sesamoids [28]. A fibrous subtalar coalition may be present in the posterior ankle, mimicking FHL tendinitis or the tarsal tunnel syndrome. This condition should be suspected when there is less than normal subtalar motion on physical examination.

The differential diagnosis of posterior ankle pain includes the following:

1. Posterior process (Shepherd's fracture) [29]
2. FHL tendinitis (dancer's tendinitis)
3. Peroneal tendinitis
4. Posterior talocalcaneal coalition
5. Posterior pseudomeniscus [4]
6. Osteoid osteoma in the posterior talus

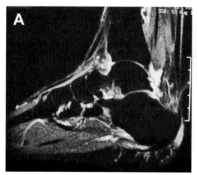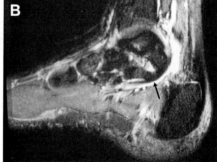

Fig. 4. (A) Fluid behind the ankle. Baker's cyst of the ankle. (B) Same ankle; fluid coming from the FHL tunnel (arrow).

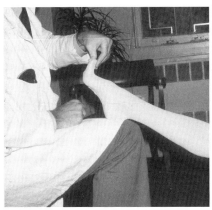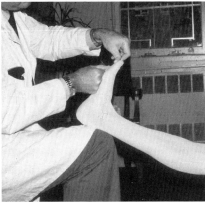

Fig. 5. Thomasen's sign. Dorsiflexion of the hallux is present when the ankle is plantar flexed (*left*) but disappears when the ankle is in dorsiflexion (*right*).

Posterior tibial tendinitis, common in athletes, is rare in dancers, an example of altered kinesiology producing altered patterns of injury. Working primarily in the equinus position produces less stress on the posterior tibial tendon but more on the FHL tendon as it passes through its pulley. In addition, dancers are selected for, and usually have, cavus feet, which are less prone to posterior tibial tendinitis. Indeed, more often than not, a dancer diagnosed with posterior tibial tendinitis on careful examination is found instead to have FHL tendinitis. Medial sprains of the ankle are rare because the medial structures are strong and rigid compared with the lateral structures. Persistent symptoms on the medial side may be caused by localized fibrous tarsal coalition of the middle facet of the Subtalar (ST) joint. This ankle also has decreased subtalar motion. Sprains of the medial ankle do occur, usually from landing off balance with sudden pronation, but this is more likely to produce a sprain of a portion of the deltoid ligament than a strain of the posterior tibial tendon. The sprain usually

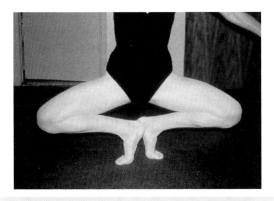

Fig. 6. A Grand Plié in fifth position; the ankle and hallux are in dorsiflexion at the same time.

affects the portion of the ligament under tension when the force was applied: the anterior deltoid if the foot was in equinus; the middle deltoid (especially the deep deltoid) if the foot was plantigrade; and the posterior portion if the foot was in dorsiflexion (rare). A stress fracture of the medial malleolus can occur but this is very rare in dancers and far more common in basketball players. An accessory bone, the os subtibiale [13], may be present in the deep portion of the deltoid; this bone can be involved in the sprain, becoming symptomatic when it had not been before. The treatment of these medial sprains and strains in the acute phase consists of the usual regimen of rest, ice, compression, and elevation; an Aircast stirrup brace; crutches if necessary; and physical therapy. A radiograph should be taken to rule out bone or physeal injury. Recovery usually is uneventful. Occasionally, a trigger point can form in the deltoid, usually around a chip fracture or accessory ossicle in the deep deltoid. These may require a corticosteroid injection if they do not respond to conservative therapy. Only rarely is surgical excision necessary. Nodules may form on the flexor digitorum longus or posterior tibial tendons following medial strains, but these usually are asymptomatic. In dancers, the most common cause of pain around the medial malleolus comes from "rolling in" (pronating) to obtain proper turnout. This produces chronic strain on the deltoid ligament, particularly the deep portion, and is one of many overuse syndromes seen in dancers. Contusion of the medial prominence of the tarsal navicular can occur. This usually happens when one foot is brought forward past the other and, as it passes the navicular, strikes the medial malleolus of the other ankle. These contusions usually heal with symptomatic treatment. On rare occasions, a fracture of the medial tubercle or disruption of an accessory navicular can occur. In this setting, the injury should be treated in a short-leg walking cast or a removable walker boot for 4 to 6 weeks to prevent the injury from becoming chronic. Strains of the spring ligament and plantar fascia can be mistaken for medial ankle pain, but a careful physical examination should make the diagnosis apparent. A rare cause of medial ankle pain is an unrecognized fracture of the colliculus located on the medial portion of the posterior tibia. This occult injury can be difficult to diagnose. It usually can be documented by a bone scan and CT scan. Another cause of medial pain just above the medial malleolus is the soleus syndrome [30,31]. This presents as chronic pain resembling a shin splint but is too far distal on the posteromedial tibial metaphysis to be a true shin splint. It is caused by an abnormal slip in the origin of the soleus muscle. The condition, similar to the exertional compartment syndrome, is much more common in athletes than dancers. It usually responds to conservative therapy, but on rare occasions release of the tight band may be necessary (Table 1).

POSTEROLATERAL ANKLE PAIN

The posterior impingement syndrome of the ankle, or talar compression syndrome [4,5,7,9,10,14,17], is the natural consequence of full weight bearing in maximum plantar flexion of the ankle in the demi-pointe or full pointe position, especially if an OT is present. It presents as posterolateral pain in the

Table 1
Differential diagnosis of medial ankle pain in athletes and dancers

Most common	Flexor hallucis longus tendonitis (dancers), posterior tibial tendonitis (athletes)
Common	Deltoid ligament sprain
Rare	Flexor digitorum longus tendonitis, soleus syndrome

back of the ankle when the posterior lip of the tibia closes against the superior border of the posterior os calcis. It can be confirmed on physical examination by tenderness behind the peroneal tendons in the back of the lateral malleolus (it often is mistaken for peroneal tendinitis); and pain with forced passive plantar flexion of the ankle, the plantar flexion sign (Fig. 7). This syndrome is often associated with an OT or trigonal process in the back of the ankle. Most people who have an OT are not aware of its presence, and the posterior impingement syndrome is rare in most athletes. It can occur in the kicking foot of a soccer player. In dancers, it may be symptomatic, and the degree of symptoms is not always related to its size. Large OTs can be minimally symptomatic and small ones sometimes can be painful. Usually the symptoms are mild and, on the whole, the OT is more often asymptomatic than symptomatic. Many world-famous ballerinas have asymptomatic OTs, and they work with them without any trouble. It is important to stress this fact to the dancer when discussing the problem, because the condition often is overdiagnosed by paramedical practitioners, who may recommend surgery unnecessarily, perhaps because of the dramatic appearance of the bone on radiograph (see Fig. 2). It is seen best on a lateral view of the ankle plantigrade and on pointe or in full plantar flexion. The diagnosis can be confirmed, if necessary, by injecting 0.5 mL of a local anesthetic into the posterolateral soft tissues behind the peroneal tendons at the superior border of the os calcis. If the pain is relieved by this injection, the diagnosis is almost certain.

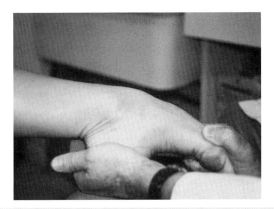

Fig. 7. The plantar flexion sign. Posterior ankle pain with forced plantar flexion.

Treatment of the posterior impingement syndrome should be graded. The first step, similar to the treatment for tendinitis, is modification of activities; nonsteroidal anti-inflammatory drugs (if the dancer is older than age 16); and physical therapy. In cases in which this approach has failed, or the symptoms recur, an injection of 0.25 to 0.5 mL of a mixture of a long-acting and a short-acting corticosteroid followed by immobilization in a removable boot for 10 to 14 days often can give dramatic and permanent relief of symptoms. This can be done accurately with the use of sonography [22]. Before injecting the steroid preparation, the clinician should confirm the diagnosis with a local anesthetic. If the local anesthetic does not relieve the symptoms, there is no point in injecting the steroids. It should be stressed that the OT usually is not a surgical problem; most dancers with an OT do not need to have it removed surgically. Occasionally, the OT does cause enough disability to warrant surgical excision but, as with most elective surgery, it is indicated only after the failure of conservative treatment in a serious dancer at least 16 years of age or older. If the problem is an isolated OT with no medial symptoms, it can be approached posterolaterally (Fig. 8) between the FHL and the peroneal tendons (with the sural nerve protected). Not infrequently, there is a combined problem of FHL tendinitis and posterior impingement. The posteromedial approach should be used in these patients (Fig. 9) so that the neurovascular bundle can be isolated and protected. A tenolysis of the FHL and removal of the adjacent OT can then be performed safely.

Other causes of posterolateral ankle pain include the following:

1. A previously asymptomatic OT may become symptomatic following an ankle sprain, resulting from disruption of its ligamentous connections and a subtle shift in position.
2. Posterior impingement can follow an ankle sprain that stretches out the lateral ligaments that hold the talus under the tibia in the relevé. As the talus moves forward, the posterior lip of the tibia comes to rest on the os calcis. The treatment for this type of posterior impingement is to tighten the lateral ankle ligaments (preferably by the Brostrom-Gould procedure) [5]. If the drawer sign can be corrected, the posterior impingement usually disappears.
3. A pseudomeniscus in posterior ankle [7] (ie, pseudomeniscal transformation of the posterior transverse ligament) can cause posterior impingement symptoms in the absence of an OT or ligament laxity. The author has seen bucket handle tears in this structure causing locking and other mechanical symptoms that are seen more often in the knee than the ankle (Tables 2 and 3).

OPERATIVE TREATMENT

Surgery is indicated when conservative therapy has failed and the symptoms warrant the risks involved in the procedure. A medial incision is indicated if the patient has a combined problem of FHL tendinitis and posterior impingement, or they have FHL tendinitis with an incidental OT that the surgeon wishes to remove along with an FHL tenolysis. The medial incision is safer

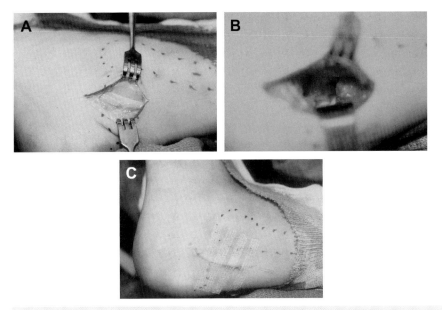

Fig. 8. (A) The posterior lateral incision. (B) The sural nerve. (C) The wound closure.

and more utilitarian because one can work safely on the lateral side from the medial approach, but it is dangerous to work medially from the lateral approach because the neurovascular bundle cannot be isolated and protected from the lateral side. The lateral approach should be used if the patient has an isolated posterior impingement without FHL tendinitis or medial symptoms. The posterior lateral clean-out can be performed with the arthroscope if one is so trained.

Tenolysis of the Flexor Hallucis Longus and Excision of the os Trigonum from the Medial Approach

Before the surgery is performed, the patient should be warned that this procedure is far better at relieving pain than improving the pointe position. If they are doing this to improve their plantar flexion, they probably will be disappointed with the result. The procedure can be performed with the patient supine because dancers usually have increased external rotation of the hip and knee that allows easy visualization of the posterior ankle from the medial side. A bloodless field is desirable, so a tourniquet is used on the thigh over cast padding. For this reason, the procedure cannot be performed with the patient under local anesthesia or ankle block. A curvilinear incision is made directly over the neurovascular bundle centered on the superior border of the os calcis (see Fig. 9A). This incision should be made carefully. The laciniate ligament lies over the neurovascular bundle but it is very thin at this level (see Fig. 9B). If the incision is made too enthusiastically, the surgeon may be in

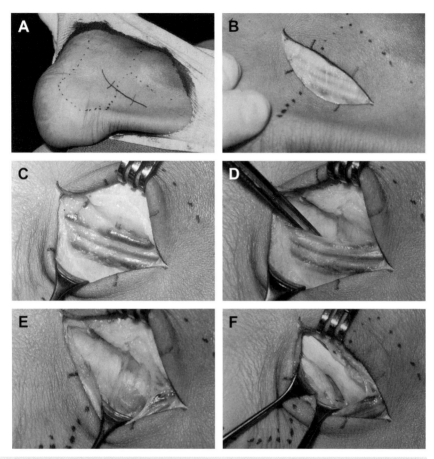

Fig. 9. (A) The posterior medial (right ankle). (B) The laciniate ligament. (C) The underlying neurovascular bundle. (D) The N-V bundle taken posteriorly. (E) The FHL sheath beneath the N-V bundle. (F) The FHL sheath opened. (G) The posterior process. (H) The posterior process excised. (I) The wound closure (in neutral dorsiflexion).

the midst of the neurovascular bundle before he or she planned. The fascia is then divided carefully to avoid damage to the artery and nerve beneath it (see Fig. 9C). At this point one must decide whether to go in front or behind the bundle. The posterior approach can take the surgeon into the variable neural branches to the os calcis. It is safer to go anterior to the bundle. All branches of the tibial nerve at this level go posterior; the safe plane is between the posterior aspect of the medial malleolus and the neurovascular bundle. The bundle can be taken down off the malleolus by blunt dissection (see Fig. 9D). Often there are several small vessels here that need to be ligated or cauterized, but once the bundle is mobilized it can be held with a blunt retractor, such as a loop or Army-Navy retractor (never with a sharp rake) (see Fig. 9E). The

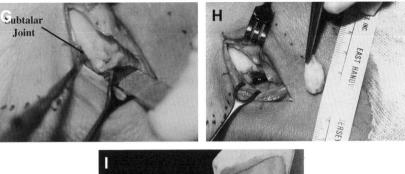

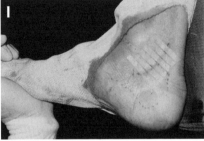

Fig. 9 (continued)

posterior tibial nerve lies directly beneath the vascular structures and is much larger than one expects, usually about the size of a pencil (see Fig. 9F). Variations in anatomy are common in this area [12,13,32]. Both the nerve and the artery divide into medial and lateral plantar branches as they leave the tarsal canal. It is not unusual for either the artery, or the nerve, or both to divide above this area, leading to reduplication within the tunnel. There also may be reduplication of the tendons (the flexor hallucis accessorius or accessory soleus muscles).

With the neurovascular bundle retracted posteriorly, the FHL is easily seen underneath the bundle by moving the hallux (see Fig. 9G). The thin fascia overlying the muscle fibers of the FHL is opened proximally, and a tenolysis is performed by opening the sheath from proximal to distal. Usually it is stenotic and tough, and the FHL often can be seen entering it at an acute angle. Care should be taken distally because the FHL tunnel and the nerve here are close together. As the tenolysis approaches the area of the sustentaculum tali,

Table 2
Flexor hallucis longus tendonitis versus posterior impingement of the ankle

Flexor hallucis longus tendonitis	Posterior impingement
Posteromedial	Posterolateral
Tenderness over flexor hallucis longus tendon	Tenderness behind fibula
Pain or triggering with motion of the hallux	Pain with plantar flexion of the ankle
Thomasen's sign [18]	Plantar flexion sign
Mistaken for posterior tibial tendonitis	Mistaken for peroneal tendonitis

Table 3
Medial versus lateral posterior ankle pain in athletes and dancers

Posteromedial	Posterolateral
Flexor hallucis longus tendonitis	Posterior impingement (os trigonum syndrome)
Posterior tibial tendonitis	Fracture trigonal process (Shepherd's fracture)
Soleus syndrome	Peroneal tendonitis
Posteromedial fibrous tarsal coalition	Pseudomeniscus syndrome

the sheath thins so that there no longer is anything to divide (see Fig. 9H). The tendon should be retracted with a blunt retractor and inspected for nodules or longitudinal tears (see Fig. 9I). Be sure to check the deep surface of the tendon because here small rents often begin. If present, these should be carefully debrided or repaired. I use a buried running stitch of 3-0 Vicryl. At this point the FHL tendon can be retracted posteriorly with the neurovascular bundle. The OT or trigonal process is found just on the lateral side of the entrance to the FHL tunnel. If the posterior aspect of the talus needs to be visualized, a capsulotomy can be performed. If there is difficulty in visualizing the OT, it helps to identify the subtalar joint (by moving the os calcis into adduction and abduction) and then follow it posteriorly; this leads to the undersurface of the OT. Once identified, it can be removed by circumferential dissection. Care should be taken to stay on the bone when performing this part of the procedure. This can be somewhat difficult, especially if the OT is large. In this case it may be necessary to remove half of the bone to gain more exposure. It is tethered laterally by the posterior talofibular ligament. Once it is removed, the posterior ankle joint should be inspected for remnants, bone fragments or loose bodies, soft tissue entrapment, or a large articular facet on the upper surface of the os calcis that articulated with the OT. If this articulation is large, it may need to be removed with a thin osteotome. The FHL sheath is not closed. The tendon does not sublux later because the direction of its pull holds the tendon in its groove. The wound then is irrigated, checked for any residual impingement by putting the foot in maximal plantar flexion while palpating the back of the ankle with a finger, and closed in layers with the ankle in neutral dorsiflexion. The patient is discharged in well-padded A-P splints for pain relief over the weekend. After a few days, weight bearing begins as tolerated with crutches as soon as possible and proceeds with swimming and physical therapy when the wound is healed. Early weight bearing is usually easier in a pair of clogs. If the FHL tendon is damaged and needs repair, the ankle is immobilized in a short-leg walking cast in neutral for 6 to 8 weeks, depending on the extent of the repair. If the tenolysis is performed without excision of the OT, recovery period is about 6 to 8 weeks. If the OT is removed along with the tenolysis, the recovery time is 8 to 12 weeks. It is important to get patients moving early to prevent stiffness. In dancers with a rather large OT, it is necessary to warn them that, once it is removed, the ankle does not just drop down into maximal plantar flexion. They must realize that the bone has been there since they were born, and removing it does not lead to immediate motion. The increased plantar flexion is obtained slowly and can be accompanied by many strange symptoms, both anteriorly and posteriorly, as the soft tissues adjust to the new range of motion.

Excision of the os Trigonum Using the Lateral Approach

Under anesthesia, the patient is placed in the lateral decubitus or prone position with a pneumatic tourniquet on thigh over cast padding. Dancers have increased external rotation of the hip; it is extremely difficult to perform this operation with the patient supine. A linear incision is made at the level of the posterior ankle mortise behind posterior border of the peroneal tendon sheath (see Fig. 8A). The sural nerve is identified in the subcutaneous tissues or carefully avoided. The dissection is carried down to the interval between the peroneal tendons laterally and the posterior ankle. Usually, the first structure seen is the posterior facet of the subtalar joint. Once this is identified, the dissection can be carried medially (see Fig. 8B) and it takes one to the undersurface of the OT or trigonal process (Stieda's process). This has attachments on all its sides: (1) superior, the posterior capsule of the talocrural joint; (2) inferior, the posterior talocalcaneal ligament, at times thick and fibrous; (3) medial, the FHL tunnel; and (4) lateral, the posterior talofibular ligament. The bone can be removed by circumferential dissection. One should be careful not to stray too far medially; the posterior tibial nerve rests directly on the medial side of the FHL tendon. The proximal entrance of the FHL tunnel can be opened if there are muscle fibers attaching distally on the FHL tendon that crowd into the tunnel when the hallux is brought into dorsiflexion (see Tomasen's sign [6]). One should not dissect medial to the FHL tendon without adequate visualization. The surgeon should check thoroughly for loose bodies; I have found them even in the FHL tunnel. The foot should be brought into maximal plantar flexion to look for any residual impingement. At times it is necessary to remove more of the posterior lateral tubercle. Often there is a facet on the upper portion of the os calcis that articulated with the OT, and this can be large enough to impinge against the posterior lip of the tibia after the OT has been removed. If necessary it also can be removed. Careful hemostasis prevents a postoperative hematoma, which can delay recovery and make early motion difficult for the patient. A layered closure then is performed with the ankle in neutral dorsiflexion. I usually close the wound with a running absorbable suture and Steri-Strips (see Fig. 8C). The patient is placed in a posterior plaster splint over the weekend and weight bearing with crutches is begun as tolerated. Early motion is essential to prevent fibrosis and resultant limited range of motion. The dancer is encouraged to swim and progress to barre exercises as discomfort subsides. Average return to full dancing is 2 to 3 months.

RESULTS

Most series reported in the literature are small. Sammarco and Miller [23] reported good results in 26 patients, a mixture of both dancers and nondancers.

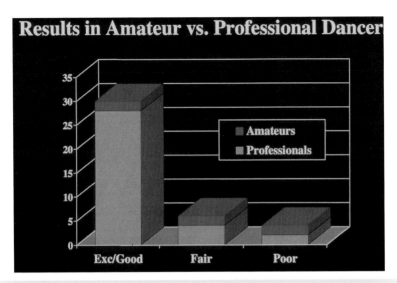

Fig. 10. The results. (*Courtesy of* W.G. Hamilton, MD, New York, NY.)

The largest series in the literature is the author's. Results were reported in 80 patients over a 10-year period. Overall results were 80% good to excellent and 20% fair to poor. The results were compared in professional versus amateur dancers and it was found that an excessive number of the fair to poor results were found in amateur dancers (Fig. 10). On the basis of this, surgeons are cautioned when operating on amateurs.

SUMMARY

Treatment of dancers can be as challenging as it is rewarding. Dancers often have unusual difficulties related to the altered kinesiology required by their individual dance form (ballet, modern dance, jazz, tap, ethnic, Broadway, and so forth). A thorough understanding of these movements helps guide the physician to the cause of the disability, particularly in the setting of overuse injuries. This knowledge, coupled with a careful physical examination, is essential for the accurate diagnosis and treatment of the dancer, who is both artist and athlete.

References
[1] Hamilton WG. Dancer's tendonitis' of the FHL tendon. Durango (CO): American Orthopedic Society for Sports Medicine; 1976.
[2] Hamilton WG. Tendonitis about the ankle joint in classical ballet dancers; dancer's tendonitis. Am J Sports Med 1977;5(2):84–8.
[3] Hamilton WG. Ballet and your body; an orthopedist's view. Dance Magazine June, July and August, 1978.
[4] Hamilton WG. Stenosing tenosynovitis of the flexor hallucis longus tendon and posterior impingement upon the os trigonum in ballet dancers. Foot Ankle 1982;3(2):74–80.
[5] Hamilton W.G. Foot and ankle injuries in dancers. In: Yokum L, editor. Sports Clinics of North America 1988;7(1):143–73.

[6] Hamilton WG. Ballet. In: Reider B, editor. The school-age athlete. Philadelphia: WB Saunders; 1991.

[7] Hamilton WG, Geppert MJ, Thompson FM. Pain in the posterior aspect of the ankle in dancers: differential diagnosis and operative treatment. J Bone Joint Surg Am 1996;78(10):1491–500.

[8] Howse AJG. Posterior block of the ankle joint in dancers. Foot Ankle 1982;3(2):81–4.

[9] Maquirrian J. Posterior ankle impingement syndrome. J Am Acad Orthop Surg 2005;13(6): 365–71.

[10] Quirk R. The talar compression syndrome in dancers. Foot Ankle 1982;3(2):65–8.

[11] Grant JCB. A method of anatomy. 5th edition. Baltimore (MD): Williams & Wilkins; 1952. p. 459, 485, 499.

[12] Hamilton WG. Surgical anatomy of the foot and ankle. Clin Symp 1985;37(3):2–32.

[13] Sarrafian SK. Anatomy of the foot and ankle. Philadelphia: JB Lippincott; 1983.

[14] Niek VD. Anterior and posterior ankle impingement. Foot Ankle Clin 2006;11(3):663–83.

[15] Thomasen E. Diseases and injuries of ballet dancers. Arhus (Denmark): Universitetsforlaget I. Arhus; 1982.

[16] Van Dijk CN. Hindfoot endoscopy for posterior ankle pain. Instr Course Lect 2006;55: 545–54.

[17] Hamilton WG, Bauam PB. Foot and ankle injuries in dancers. In: Coughlin MJ, Mann RA, Saltzman JJ, editors. Surgery of the foot and ankle. Philadelphia: Abelex; 2006. p. 1223–4.

[18] Keeling JJ, Guyton GP. Endoscopic flexor hallucis longus decompression: a cadaver study. Foot Ankle Int 2007;28(7):810–4.

[19] Kolettis GJ, Micheli LJ, Klein JD. Release of the flexor hallucis longus tendon in ballet dancers. J Bone Joint Surg Am 1996;78(9):1386–90.

[20] Lui TH. Arthroscopy and endoscopy of the foot and ankle: indications for new techniques. Arthroscopy 2007;23(8):889–902.

[21] Mulier T, Rummens E, Dereymaeker G. Risk of neurovascular injuries in flexor hallucis longus tendon transfers: an anatomic cadaver study. Foot Ankle Int 2007;28(8):910–5.

[22] Mehdizade A, Adler RS. Sonographically guided flexor hallucis longus tendon sheath injection. J Ultrasound Med 2007;26(2):233–7.

[23] Sammarco JG, Miller EH. Partial rupture of the flexor hallucis longus tendon in classical ballet dancers: two case reports. J Bone Joint Surg Am 1979;61(1):149–50.

[24] Sammarco JG, Cooper PS. Flexor hallucis longus tendon injury in dancers and non-dancers. Foot Ankle Int 1998;19(6):356–62.

[25] Romash MM. Closed rupture of the flexor hallucis longus tendon in a long distance runner: report of a case and review of the literature. Foot Ankle Int 1994;15(8):433–6.

[26] SY Wei, Kneeland JB, Okereke E. Complete atraumatic rupture of the flexor hallucis longus tendon: a case report and review of the literature. Foot Ankle Int 1998;19(7):472–4.

[27] Boruta A, Tiemann A, Richter J, et al. Partial tear of the flexor hallucis longus at the knot of Henry: presentation of three cases. Foot Ankle Int 1997;18(4):243–6.

[28] Sanhudo JA. Stenosing tenosynovitis of the flexor hallucis longus tendon at the sesamoid area. Foot Ankle Int 2002;23(9):801–3.

[29] Shepherd FJ. A hitherto undescribed fracture of the astragalus. J Anat Physiol 1882;17:79.

[30] Michael RH, Holder LE. The soleus syndrome. Am J Sports Med 1985;13(2):87–94.

[31] Michelson J, Dunn L. Tenosynovitis of the flexor hallucis longus: a clinical study of the spectrum of presentation and treatment. Foot Ankle Int 2005;26(4):291–303.

[32] Eberle CF, Moran B, Gleason T. The accessory flexor digitorum longus as a cause of Flexor Hallucis Syndrome. Foot Ankle Int 2002;23(1):51–5.

Clin Sports Med 27 (2008) 279–288

CLINICS IN SPORTS MEDICINE

ELSEVIER
SAUNDERS

Tendon Injuries in Dance

Christopher W. Hodgkins, MD[a], John G. Kennedy, MD, MMSc, MCh, FRCSI, FRCS (Orth)[b,*], Padhraigh F. O'Loughlin, MD[b]

[a]Department of Orthopaedic Surgery, University of Miami, Miller School of Medicine, Jackson Memorial Hospital, Ryder Trauma Center, P.O. Box 016960 (D-27), Miami, FL 33101, USA
[b]Hospital for Special Surgery, 523 East 72nd Street, Suite 514, New York, NY, 10021, USA

Professional ballet dancers require an extraordinary anatomic, physiologic, and psychologic makeup to achieve and sustain their level of ability and activity. Although many attempt to attain this, very few have all the ingredients necessary. Those that do graduate to this elite corps are then subject to a myriad of injuries as a result of the extreme demands of this profession.

Tendon injuries are common in the dancers' profession. Many are secondary to poor technique, inappropriate training and performance and unfavorable intrinsic factors. They often coexist with other pathologies of the bone, ligaments and psyche. It is critical therefore that the dance doctor does not examine the tendon injury in isolation. Before discussing tendon injuries and treatment strategies it is essential first to understand the basics of their anatomy, histology, and pathologic processes.

TENDON STRUCTURE

Tendons transmit forces between muscle and bone. Their basic makeup consists of collagen bundles that provide tensile strength, cells, and extracellular matrix or ground substance. The ground substance provides structural support for the collagen and regulates its formation from procollagen. Tenocytes are found sparsely among collagen fibers and synthesize the ground substance and procollagen [1]. The more complex structure is beyond the scope of this article.

The tendon is covered by a fine loose connective tissue layer, the epitenon, which contains the vascular, lymphatic and nerve supply. Superficial to this is the paratenon, a loose areolar connective tissue consisting of type I and III collagen [1,2].

*Corresponding author. E-mail address: kennedyj@hss.edu (J.G. Kennedy).

0278-5919/08/$ – see front matter
doi:10.1016/j.csm.2007.12.003

TERMINOLOGY

Pathologic terminology is based on histologic findings and is often used incorrectly in a clinical setting leading to incorrect treatment strategies. Tendinopathy is an umbrella term encompassing a range of pathologies considered to be part of the same spectrum from tendonitis (acute microscopic inflammation of the tendon) to paratenonitis (acute inflammation of the paratenon layer) to tendinosis (chronic intrasubstance tendon degeneration) to the end stage of partial or complete rupture (Box 1).

INJURY RESPONSE

The typical histologic response to acute tendon injury consists of an inflammatory, proliferative, and maturation stage. Cell mobilization in the inflammatory stage lasts approximately 48 hours. Many proteolytic enzymes exist during this phase and it is essential to limit this period before collagen repair can begin. Ground substance facilitates formation of insoluble collagen, which progresses to insoluble immature collagen. Organization of collagen fibrils occurs during the maturation phase and is influenced by Wolff's law according to the direction of the tensile forces in the structure. It remains unclear how much tensile force is optimal for this [3].

TENDON INJURIES

Thirteen tendons pass the ankle, all of which are subject to potential injury. There is a distinct collection and pattern of injuries, however, to which professional dancers are susceptible. This is true for many sports and is dependent on the individual stresses endured during activity. The etiology of these injuries can be acutely traumatic, dance related, or otherwise, and is typically more commonly chronic. Chronic injuries can be secondary to overuse, intrinsic abnormalities, and extrinsic factors.

Basic Examination of the Dancer

Begin by examining the athlete as they walk into the clinic. Examine the footwear before uncovering both lower extremities. Inspect alignment and arches recumbent, weight bearing, and in relevé. Inspect for skin changes, erythema,

---

Box 1: Basic definitions

Tendonitis: Implies acute histologic inflammation in the substance of the tendon. Clinically acute and symptomatic.

Tendonosis: Implies intratendonous degeneration, collagen disorientation, increase in mucoid ground substance with resultant loss of normal collagen architecture. Lack of acute inflammatory cells. Can be clinically asymptomatic. More often associated with rupture, partial or complete.

Paratendonitis: Acute inflammation of the surrounding tendon sheath. Clinically symptomatic.

previous scars, and focal swelling. Palpate for areas of tenderness and calluses. Range the joints and examine the extraordinary arcs of movement. Identify pain at extremes of movement. Test for anterior draw and stress for instability. Have the athlete toe walk and heel walk.

To identify specific tendon pathology have the dancer actively resist forceful resistance of plantar flexion, dorsiflexion, and inversion and eversion throughout the range of flexion at the ankle. This often triggers pain, which can be specifically located with careful palpation.

As an added examination point it is important to assess the general physical and mental health of the dancer. Although the identification of and certainly treatment of such issues is not the role of the orthopedic surgeon, they adversely affect the outcome of treatment. Referral to the appropriate specialist leads to an overall more satisfactory outcome. Examining the athlete's demeanor and responses to diagnosis explanations and treatment suggestions can often indicate their trust and compliance tendencies.

Obtain plain anteroposterior, lateral, and mortise views of the ankle and anteroposterior, lateral, and oblique views of the foot as necessary. It may be necessary to obtain radiographs in relevé to identify specific pathologies, especially osseous impingements.

The following addresses the more common tendonopathies, focusing on their individual anatomy, function, injury patterns, and treatment.

ACHILLES TENDON

The Achilles tendon is a common site for injury in the dancer. It must transmit up to six times body weight during running and jumping [4]. The Achilles tendon arises from the gastrocnemius-soleus complex. The medial and lateral heads of the gastrocnemius muscle take origin from posterior aspect of respective femoral condyles. The soleus muscle originates from the tibia and fibula. The tendon inserts on the posterior aspect of the calcaneus.

Many factors can contribute to Achilles injury including tight heel chords, small or thin tendon mass, pronation or "rolling in," incomplete relevé, and a cavus foot with Haglund's deformity [4,5].

Acute Tendinitis

This is a common presentation and can be limited to the tendon or involve the surrounding paratenon (Fig. 1). Distinction can be made on examination. Peritendonitis is characterized by crepitus, exquisite tenderness, and swelling that does not move with the tendon. Examination of a chronic tendonosis reveals an absence of crepitation and swelling, often with focal tender nodules that move as the ankle is plantar and dorsiflexed.

Generic Approach to Initial Treatment of Tendonitis

Treatment of acute tendonitis or paratendonosis should follow a two-stage regimen. Firstly, insist on the protocol of strict rest, immobilization, cold, and elevation in combination with oral anti-inflammatory medication if tolerated. It is absolutely imperative to halt the cycle of inflammation that has resulted from

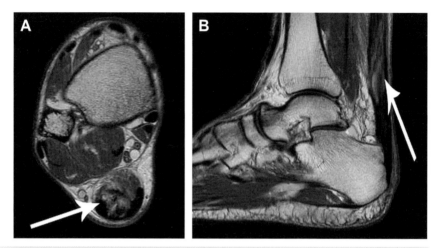

Fig. 1. Axial (A) and sagital (B) plane MRI demonstrating a degenerated Achilles tendon (arrow).

acute microtears and irritation of the tendon or its enveloping sheath. This is achieved by strict immobilization in a Cam boot for 23 hours per day for an initial period of 2 weeks followed by re-examination. If clinically the inflammation and tenderness has settled the second stage of treatment can begin with a very gentle controlled stretching regimen to restore length and strength to the tendon. This is ideally delivered by a therapist familiar with dance to obtain an optimal outcome. Steroid injections should be avoided in the professional dancer because their relationship to decreasing long-term tendon strength and association with late rupture is still unclear [6]. It is also important to identify and correct predisposing factors before they become repeat offenders and also institute preventative measures, such as the use of stretch boxes before and during performances.

Under no circumstances should nonsteroidal anti-inflammatory drugs be used to allow the dancer to function for performances. It is not infrequent, given personal and professional pressure, to find dancers not following treatment protocols to perform. In such cases it may be necessary to immobilize these individuals in a cast to ensure compliance.

Care must be taken to consider carefully the possibility of other sources of pain in this region as either the sole contributing cause or as concurrent pathologies that must also be addressed to avoid delay in treatment. Common pathologies are retrocalcaneal bursitis, os trigonum impingement, os trigonum fracture, and flexor hallucis longus (FHL) tendonosis. It is beyond the scope of this article to address these in detail.

Achilles Tendonosis

Chronic Achilles tendon pathology can be the long-term result of multiple episodes of acute tendonitis resulting in mucoid degenerative changes (Fig. 2).

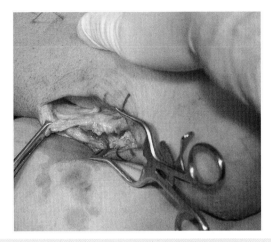

Fig. 2. Intraoperative photograph of a degenerated Achilles tendon.

Clinically, it may be asymptomatic but if not it requires intervention. A similar strategy to that used for acute flare-up can be trialed as a first measure. Definitive treatment may require surgical repair, excision of nodules, removal of fibrotic adhesions, and debridement of degenerative tissue. The tendon is repaired with absorbable suture. Postoperatively the patient is immobilized in 20 degrees of plantar flexion for 2 weeks followed by 10 degrees for a further 2 weeks and then placed in removable Cam boot for a final 2 weeks of immobilization [7]. Gentle supervised stretching exercises can then begin.

Achilles Tendon Rupture

Rupture is most often the end result of chronic degenerative changes in the tendon. It most commonly occurs in male dancers over the age of 30. Clinically, it presents as acute pain and swelling. The Thompson test is positive.

The ability to plantar flex the foot does not rule out this injury because the posterior tibial tendon and the toe flexors can contribute to this motion. Similarly, the lack of palpable defect in the tendon because of hematoma formation can fool the examiner.

In the professional dancer open surgical repair is the preferred treatment method. The aim of the procedure is to restore the tendon to length to maximize potential return to normal strength. This can be done by primary repair or with augmentation using the plantaris tendon. Preparing the contralateral lower leg into the field allows more accurate estimation of anatomic tendon length [4,7,8].

PERONEAL TENDONS

The pernoei originate from the anterolateral surface of the proximal two thirds of the fibula. The brevis tendon inserts into the base of the fifth metatarsal and the longus tendon inserts on to the plantar surface of the medial cuneiform and base of the first metatarsal. The retrofibular pace in which the tendons lie is a shallow groove on the posterolateral surface of the distal fibula. The brevis tendon sits anteriorly in contact with the groove, whereas the longus sits behind the groove. The tendons are restricted in this groove by the superior peroneal retinaculum. Tendons can sublux out of this groove in a habitual or traumatic manner. Traumatic subluxations require surgical repair. The provocative maneuver thought to be responsible for traumatic subluxation is a sudden forceful dorsiflexion in a position of slight inversion [3–9].

The peronei function as strong everters, weak plantar flexors, and are the primary lateral dynamic stabilizers of the ankle. The cavovarus foot that many dancers have predisposes to a tendency for peroneal tendinopathy rather than posterior tibial tendon pathology.

Peroneal pathology occurs in dancers but is far less common than in other athletes. Aggravation of peroneus longus can occur as it passes the cuboid in the foot. This is more common in association with an os peronei. Care must be taken to avoid misdiagnosis because subluxation of the cuboid and other retrocalcaneal pathologies can present similarly and in conjunction. Peroneal pathology is thought often to be secondary to chronic lateral ankle instability and this must not be missed when treating the latter [7].

Treatment of peroneal tendonitis (Fig. 3) follows the same regimen described previously. A lateral heel wedge in the Cam boot can help off-load the tendons. Surgical debridement for chronic symptomatology can be performed but is rarely indicated. More commonly procedures to address lateral ankle ligament instability and peroneal subluxations are required. Rupture of the peroneal tendons although rare can occur and most commonly occurs at the cuboid notch [10].

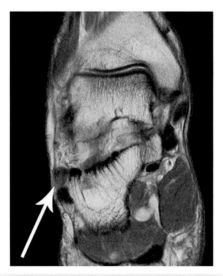

Fig. 3. Coronal plane MRI demonstrating a chronic peroneus brevis incomplete tear (arrow).

POSTERIOR TIBIAL TENDON

The posterior tibialis muscle takes origin for the proximal intramuscular septum in the calf and its tendon passes posterior and medial to the ankle in the tarsal tunnel and inserts in a broad fashion into the naviculum, cuneiforms, and bases of the middle three metatarsals. It is a plantar flexor and inverter of the foot.

Pathology affecting the posterior tibialis tendon is also less common in dancers than standard professional athletes given their protective cavovarus anatomy. It is more often the flexor hallucis longus that is injured in dancers with pain in the medial ankle [4].

Treatment of posterior tibial tendonitis (Fig. 4) should follow the regimen discussed previously. A medial heel wedge in the boot can aid in offloading the tendon somewhat. Chronic and recurrent pathology may require surgical intervention in the form of tenolysis as described previously to debride degenerative tendon and mucoid substance with primary suture repair [7].

FLEXOR HALLUCIS LONGUS

The flexor hallucis longus has been called the Achilles tendon of the foot and is so frequently injured that it has become known as "dancer's tendonitis" [4]. The flexor hallucis longus takes origin from the middle posterior third of the fibula and inserts into the plantar base of the distal phalanx. Around the ankle it passes through a fibrosseous tunnel behind the talus between the medial and lateral tubercles.

It is through this fibrosseous tunnel that it often becomes compromised. Like a rope in a pulley the tendon becomes frayed, which causes swelling and

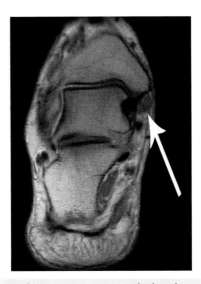

Fig. 4. Coronal plane MRI demonstrating posterior tibial tendonosis (arrow).

microtears. This in turn causes more aggravation in the narrow tunnel and a vicious cycle ensues. If left untreated a nodule or partial tear inevitably develops.

The presence of a nodule, or obstruction, to a smooth passage through the fibrosseous tunnel causes triggering (Fig. 5). This is known as "hallux saltans." Rarely, the tendon can become frozen in its sheath causing a pseudo hallux rigidus [4,7].

Dancers who perform repetitive push-off from the forefoot and spend time in en-pointe and demi-pointe and grand-plie positions predispose themselves to this condition (Fig. 6).

Treatment consists of the standard approach described previously. It is essential to emphasize that rest is the vital ingredient in addition to nonsteroidal anti-inflammatory drugs, ice and physical therapy. Using these modalities without rest to allow further participation only leads to further damage.

Persistent and recurrent episodes of flexor hallucis longus tendonitis may require surgical tenolysis but only after failure of well-executed conservative therapy. Postoperative rehabilitation sidelines the dancer for at least 3 months [7]. Flexor hallucis longus tendontitis can also occur at Henry's knot or as it passes between the sesamoids under the head of the first metatarsal, although much less frequently than at the ankle.

OTHER TENDINOPATHIES

The following pathologies are rare in dancers and follow the same treatment regimens already described. The anterior tibial tendon takes origin from the proximal two thirds of the tibia, lateral tibial condyle, and the interosseous membrane. Its tendon runs through the anterior tarsal tunnel and inserts onto the plantar-medial first cuneiform and first metatarsal. Primary function is dorsiflexion. Its excursion is constricted by superior and inferior retinaculi. It's straight course and absence of a bony fulcrum makes it less susceptible to aggravation.

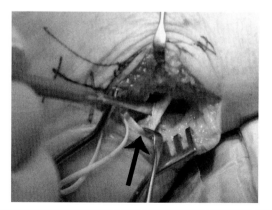

Fig. 5. Intraoperative photograph demonstrating a torn fibrotic flexor hallucis longus (*arrow*).

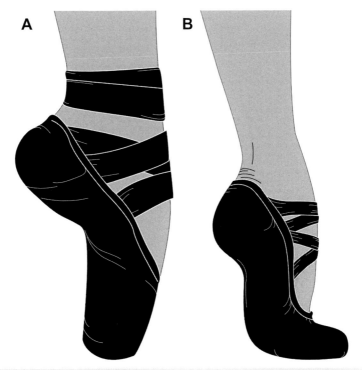

Fig. 6. Illustration of the en-pointe (A) and demi-pointe (B) positions.

Pathology of the extensor digitorum longus and extensor hallucis longus is rare for the same reasons as those mentioned for the anterior tibial tendon, because they follow a very similar proximal course.

SUMMARY

Dancers by nature have very unique anatomy, training, and performance requirements and mentalities. All of these factors contribute to a very unique set of pathologies and difficult treatment approaches. It is very important to understand the technicality and physicality of ballet to approach and address problems. Careful educated examination and consideration guide one to the existing or coexisting pathologies and allow targeted treatment. It is essential that this treatment be delivered correctly and that compliance be achieved. With these factors in mind expedient and successful return to training and performance should follow.

References
  [1] Maffulli N, Wong J, Almedkinders LC. Types and epidemiology of tendinopathy. Clin Sports Med 2003;22(4):675–92.
  [2] Khan K, Cook J. The painful non ruptured tendon: clinical aspects. Clin Sports Med 2003;22(4):711–25.

[3] Frey CC, Shereff MJ. Tendon injuries about the ankle in athletes. Clin Sports Med 1988;7(1):103–18.

[4] Hamilton WG. Foot and ankle injuries in dancers. Clin Sports Med 1988;7(1):143–73.

[5] Scheller AD, Kasser JR, Quigley TB. Tendon injuries about the ankle. Clin Sports Med 1983;2(3):631–41.

[6] Wilder RP, Sethi S. Overuse injuries: tendinopathies, stress fractures, compartment syndrome, and shin splints. Clin Sports Med 2004;23(1):55–81.

[7] Kennedy JG, Hodgkins CW, Columbier J-A, et al. Foot and ankle injuries in dancers. International SportMed Journal 2007;8(No.3):141–65. Available at: http://www.ismj.com. Accessed December 2007.

[8] Brown TD, Micheli LJ. Foot and ankle injuries in dance. Am J Orthop 2004;33(6):303–9.

[9] Macintyre J, Joy E. Foot and ankle injuries in dance. Clin Sports med 2000;19(2):351–68.

[10] Selmani E, Gjata V, Gjika E. Current concepts review: peroneal tendon disorders. Foot Ankle Int 2006;27(3):221–8.

Clin Sports Med 27 (2008) 289–294

CLINICS IN SPORTS MEDICINE

Posterior Tibial Tendon Tears in Dancers

Jonathan T. Deland, MD[a],*, William G. Hamilton, MD[b]

[a]Foot and Ankle Service, Hospital for Special Surgery, 535 East 70th Street, New York, NY 10021, USA
[b]Orthopaedic Associates of New York, 343 West 58th Street, New York, NY 10019, USA

osterior tibial tendon tears in dancers are uncommon [1]. No case series of such injuries has been presented. The injury does however occur, and should be differentiated from the more common causes of medial hindfoot symptoms in dancers. The relevant anatomy, biomechanics, and differential diagnosis are presented followed by a summary of four cases.

ANATOMY OF BIOMECHANICS

After originating from the posterior proximal tibia, the posterior tibial tendon muscle courses along the posterior and medial aspect of the tibia with the tendon proceeding around the medial malleolus to insert on the navicular as well as the middle three metatarsal bases and cuneiforms. Its course around the medial malleolus constitutes a stress riser for the tendon and is also a zone of hypovascularity. Because the posterior tibial tendon has the greatest mechanical advantage to invert the foot and thereby lock the triple joint complex, it is an important contributor for the foot's ability to become a rigid lever for the heel rise [2,3]. It provides a critical function in the foot and is, therefore, very important in athletes. It suffers the greatest strain most probably in a flatfoot and during gait when the foot is flat and the muscle is under eccentric contraction or attempting heel rise. Once heel rise has occurred, the geometry of the joints help in stability. Dancers have exceptional proprioception and balance to enable them to go up on point. They are a selected group with a foot that easily and efficiently achieves heel rise and often have a higher arch foot than a flatter one. It is, therefore, not surprising that dancers are not particularly prone to posterior tibial tendon injuries. However, as in young athletes, the tendon still may be injured, and it is important for a dancer just as other athletes, that the injury be recognized and treated properly.

*Corresponding author. E-mail address: delandj@hss.edu (J.T. Deland).

0278-5919/08/$ – see front matter
doi:10.1016/j.csm.2007.12.001

CLASSIC POSTERIOR TIBIAL TENDON INSUFFICIENCY AND POSTERIOR TIBIAL TENDON INJURY TO THE YOUNG ATHLETE

Classic posterior tibial tendon insufficiency often is an insidious degeneration of the tendon that does not present with an acute incident [2–4]. The patient notes medial pain over the tendon inferior and distal to the medial malleolus. Most commonly, there is a pre-existing flatfoot from which further deformity develops. The treatment not only involves treating the degenerating tendon but the often progressive deformity as well. The deformity includes increased heel valgus and abduction through the talonavicular joint and may involve the more distal joints as well.

The injury to the young athlete, such as a dancer, is usually quite different [5]. Although it can be associated with a flatfoot, it is not necessarily so. Most often it is an acute injury, from a sudden overload of the tendon. Because the flatfoot is not necessarily the etiology, the bony procedures to realign the arch may not be necessary. Also, procedures such as a calcaneal osteotomy may certainly negatively impact the performance of a dancer. The use of a flexor digitorum tendon transfer in a dancer who depends on toe function is likely to negatively impact toe flexion and thereby the dancer's ability to perform necessary movements for dance.

DIAGNOSIS

The diagnosis of posterior tibial tendon tear is not difficult. If the examiner knows how to palpate the tendon, tenderness over the tendon can be easily confirmed (Fig. 1). Tensioning the tendon by having the patient invert and plantarflex the foot should be done, and tenderness directly over tendon inferior to the medial malleolus can be confirmed. The patient most often will have discomfort or possibly difficulty with single stance heel rise. The presence of a tear should be

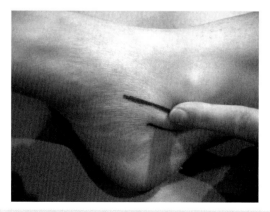

Fig. 1. Medial aspect of the ankle. Finger points to location of posterior tibial tendon (upper line). Lower line is the level of the FHL.

confirmed by an experienced ultrasonographer or MRI radiologist. On a properly done MRI scan, a split or tear of the posterior tibial tendon can be seen on axial images most commonly at or inferior to the medial malleolus.

DIFFERENTIAL DIAGNOSIS

The posterior tibial tendon injury must be differentiated from other possible causes of medial pain in dancers [6]. In a dancer, a more common cause of medial pain is flexor hallucis longus (FHL) tenosynovitis and posterior impingement [7]. The medial tenderness will be centered on the FHL inferior and just proximal to the sustentaculum tali not at the posterior tibial tendon. By palpating the posterior tibial tendon when the foot is inverted and plantar flexed, the examiner can differentiate the location of the posterior tibial tendon from that of the FHL. The flexor hallucis longus tendon is more inferior (plantar) to that of the posterior tibial tendon.

A young athlete can have pain radiating along medial distal tibia down to the level of the medial malleolus. Although this could be from a partial tear of the posterior tibial tendon at this level, it is more common to be from other conditions. A medial tibial stress fracture should be excluded and can be identified by more tenderness directly over the bone than over the tendon. If necessary, a bone scan can be used to confirm the diagnosis. More uncommon is the soleus syndrome [8]. In this condition there is tenderness at the soleus fascia insertion on the medial border of the tibia proximal to the medial malleolus and adjacent to the posterior tibial tendon. With an experienced radiologist or ultrasonographer, the posterior tibial tendon can be shown to be normal at this level in the condition. If conservative treatments fail, release of the soleus fascia can give dramatic relief of pain.

CASE REVIEWS OF POSTERIOR TIBIAL TENDON TEARS IN DANCERS

There is little in the literature on the subject of posterior tibial tendon tears in dancers. An informal survey of the two major New York City–based Ballet Companies in America (The New York City Ballet and American Ballet Theatre) plus their associated schools confirm this statement. The reason for this is speculative, but it is probably because of the cavus foot for which most dancers are selected. In many ways, the posterior tibial tendon is protected by the cavus foot because it is difficult to pronate this foot and strain the tendon. The senior author has seen several cases of acute dislocation of the posterior tibial tendon in dancers, but even in these patients the tendon itself was undamaged. Tendonitis around the posterior medial ankle in a dancer almost always involves the FHL tendon in its sheath and is so common it is called "dancer's tendonitis" [7].

Interestingly, there currently is a trend in professional ballet dancers to cross-train for conditioning. Any posterior tibial tendonitis that has been seen in these companies has occurred as a result of the cross-training workouts in the gym rather than the dance rehearsals and performances themselves. On rare occasions the tendon can become irritated because of a direct blow or contusion, but in this younger population it usually heals uneventfully.

With this in mind, after 30 years of not seeing any problems other than 3 acute dislocations with no damage to the posterior tibial tendon t'ndon, we subsequently have seen four severe injuries in professional dancers, three of which required surgery with long recoveries. One healed with prolonged immobilization. Fortunately, all have returned to their professional careers.

- AH, a 24-year-old professional ballet dancer (corps) had pain in the right ankle without specific trauma. It was treated conservatively but failed to heal. She had a cavus foot with no pronation. Surgery revealed a partial tear of the tendon at the level of the retinaculum. The tendon was repaired, and the patient returned to dancing 9 months later.
- KJ, a 29-year-old Radio City Music Hall (Rockette) dancer landed off balance in a rehearsal and had pain in the retinacular area of the right posterior tibial tendon. MRI and sonogram showed a partial tear at this level. She had a moderately cavus foot with no pronation. She was treated in a CAM walker with a heel lift and medial wedge for 6 weeks then in clogs and swimming. Rehabilitation with resisted exercises and stretching were not begun until 12 weeks after injury. She was pain free and ready to return at the professional level 5 months after her injury.
- JS, a 31-year-old professional ballerina landed off balance injuring the left posterior tibial tendon. She tried to dance with the pain and sustained a further episode of severe sharp pain. She had a moderately cavus foot with no pronation. A workup revealed "partial tear with degeneration." Conservative therapy failed and surgical exploration revealed a severe tear and degeneration from the musculotendinous junction to the insertion in the navicular (Fig. 2). Approximately 25% to 30% of the tendon was unrepairable and was debrided. The remaining 70% was repaired and retubularized (Fig. 3). An Flexor Digitorum Longus (FDL) graft was not performed for fear that weakness in her lesser toes would inhibit her balance later on demi-pointe.

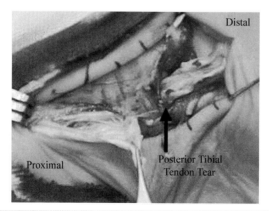

Fig. 2. Posterior tibial tendon tear in a dancer located inferior to the sheath left intact at the medial malleolus.

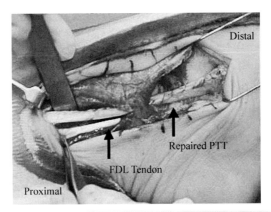

Fig. 3. Repaired posterior tibial tendon with repair distal and at the level of the medial malleolus (intact sheath).

Recovery was very slow to give the repaired tendon plenty of time to heal. Physical therapy was not begun until 3 to 4 months postoperatively and progressed very slowly. She returned to full dancing 13 months after her surgery and has continued to work at 90% function 3 years after her injury. We have been very careful to protect this dancer and will not allow her to be cast in major roles on consecutive nights.

- PV, a 31-year-old professional ballet dancer sustained a "minor strain" of her left posterior tibial tendon, which failed to heal in spite of cast immobilization. She also had a moderately cavus foot without pronation. Exploration found a tear at the level of the retinaculum. It was debrided and repaired above and below the retinaculum without taking it down. Again, plenty of time was allowed for healing, and therapy was not begun for 3 months after surgery. She retuned to full dancing 6 months later but complained of some mild stiffness.

These cases have some unifying characteristics. They were all associated with an acute injury or strain. Some cases were thought initially not to be serious. They occurred more proximal and closer to the medial malleolus than many of the cases of posterior tibial tendon insufficiency where the tears can be closer to the navicular attachment. They do not seem to be associated with a flatfoot or pronation. Based on experience in this small number of cases, the following recommendations can be given. Success can be obtained with debridement and repair. The recovery is long, but a calcaneal osteotomy or FDL transfer is not necessary.

SUMMARY

Posterior tibial tendon injuries are rare in dancers but do occur. They should be differentiated from more common medial "ankle" injuries in dancers, such as FHL tenosynovitis. The injury is different from that in posterior tibial tendon insufficiency which is a slow degenerative process associated with a flatfoot. Success in these more acute injuries in dancers can be obtained with debridement and repair followed by slow rehabilitation.

References

[1] Macintyre J, Joy E. Foot and ankle injuries in dance. The Athletic Woman 2000;19(2): 351–68.

[2] Deland JT. Foot and ankle: tendon disorders. In: Lin SS, Berberian WS, editors. Orthopedic surgery essentials. Philadelphia: Lippincott, Williams, and Wilkins; 2004. p. 153–81.

[3] Deland JT. Posterior Tibial Tendon Dysfunction. In: Edward V. Craig, editor. Clinical Orthopaedics. Philadelphia: Lippincott, Williams, and Wilkins; 1999. p. 883–91.

[4] Deland JT, Page A, Sung I, et al. Posterior tibial tendon insufficiency results at different stages. HSS Journal 2006;2(2):157–60.

[5] Conti SF. Posterior tibial tendon problems in athletes. Orthop Clin North Am 1994;25(1): 109–21.

[6] Hamilton WG, Bauman JH. Foot and ankle injury in dancers. In: Coughlin MJ, Mann RA, Saltzman CL, editors. Surgery of the foot and ankle. Philadelphia: Mosby Elsevier; 2007. p. 1603–40.

[7] Hamilton WG. Stenosing tenosynovitis of the flexor hallucis longus tendon and posterior impingement upon the os trigonum in ballet dancers. Foot Ankle 1982;3(2):74–80.

[8] Michael RH, Holder LE. The soleus syndrome: a cause of medial tibial stress (shin splints). Am J Sports Med 1985;13(2):87–94.

Clin Sports Med 27 (2008) 295–304

CLINICS IN SPORTS MEDICINE

ELSEVIER
SAUNDERS

Foot and Ankle Fractures in Dancers

Megan Goulart, BS[a], Martin J. O'Malley, MD[a,b],
Christopher W. Hodgkins, MD[c], Timothy P. Charlton, MD[d],*

[a]Weill Medical College of Cornell University, 523 East 72nd Street, New York, NY 10021, USA
[b]Hospital for Special Surgery, 523 East 72nd Street, New York, NY 10021, USA
[c]Department of Orthopaedic Surgery, University of Miami, Miller School of Medicine, Jackson
Memorial Hospital, Ryder Trauma Center, P.O. Box 016960 (D-27), Miami, FL 33101, USA
[d]Keck School of Medicine, University of Southern California, 1520 San Pablo Street, Suite 2000,
Los Angeles, CA 90023, USA

The intense physical demands of dancing put dancers at high risk for numerous injuries to the foot and ankle. These injuries, in terms of fractures, fall into three general categories: overuse or stress fractures, acute traumatic fractures, and an acute fracture in the setting of an underlying chronic stress injury. Acute injuries can be from a single instance of overstress or from a traumatic episode and often result from loss of balance during a jump or a fatigue event. When fatigued, dancers often fail to gain adequate height during jumps and land incorrectly. A lack of adequate stabilization due to weakness and fatigue of the peroneal musculature can also result in acute injuries. When the foot or ankle is forced beyond its natural maximum range of motion, acute fractures and other bony impaction injuries can occur.

Stress injuries are common secondary to repetitive mictrotrauma to bony, ligamentous, and musculotendinous structures. They often result when the body is unable to absorb the forces generated by the repeated cyclic loading of musculoskeletal structures. Although dancers are susceptible to injury due to the physical nature of their profession, a number of other intrinsic and extrinsic factors contribute to the high injury rate. The biomechanical demands of dance; a dancer's training methods, shoes, and dance surfaces; a dancer's overall fitness, strength, flexibility, and alignment; variations in bony and ligamentous structures; and a dancer's nutritional and hormonal status all contribute to osseous insult and injury recovery. Additional factors include inappropriate training methods, excessive duration and intensity of training, failure to allow sufficient adaptation time to new training levels, and failure to allow for adequate recovery from activity and injury.

Whether a dancer dances more or less than 5 hours daily is a great predictor of injury level. When dancers' muscles are fatigued, their technical mechanics break down and they lose the protective capacity to prevent injury [1]. Muscles,

*Corresponding author. E-mail address: timothy.charlton@usc.edu (T.P. Charlton).

0278-5919/08/$ – see front matter
doi:10.1016/j.csm.2008.01.002

ligaments, tendons, and bones are overloaded and therefore more vulnerable to injury. The female athlete triad of disordered eating, amenorrhea, and low bone density also greatly increases a female dancer's propensity to bony injury while dancing.

CLINICAL PRESENTATION AND ASSESSMENT

A dancer's acute inability to bear weight on a painful extremity is suggestive of an acute fracture; however, presentations may be much more subtle than this, and a careful history of the dancer's symptoms and dance history is always necessary to avoid missing essential information. Meticulous physical examination guides the physician to selective radiographic assessment and differential diagnosis. It is especially important not to overlook proximal fifth metatarsal injuries and fractures of the medial or lateral dome of the talus, lateral process of the talus, os trigonum, and anterior process of the calcaneus. In adolescent dancers, soft-tissue swelling over the physis is often suggestive of an epiphyseal fracture, which can be subtle. Also important is that clinical symptoms from stress fractures may precede radiographic findings by many weeks.

Chronic foot pain unresponsive to conventional treatment is often due to an occult fracture of the tarsal bones. Persistent deep ankle pain, ankle effusions, and catching or a loose sensation within the ankle can be the result of osteochondral injuries of the talus. Clinical situations such as these warrant further investigation using CT with or without MRI as necessary to confirm diagnosis. Clinical and radiologic assessment must consider osseous, ligamentous, and tendon pathology. Selective local anesthetic injection can be invaluable in identifying the true source of pain in difficult cases.

GENERIC TREATMENT STRATEGY OF FRACTURES

Although differences occur in the exact management of the individual fractures considered here, a generic treatment protocol exists. Specific deviations from this protocol for the individual fractures described are mentioned as necessary.

All fractures require immediate rest, immobilization, cold, and elevation. Avoidance of the precipitating activity is essential. The type and length of immobilization is controversial but certain principles must be followed. Cam boots are removable and therefore not suitable for patients who you suspect will be noncompliant. Because noncompliance is high in the dancing profession due to internal and external pressure to return to training and performance, casting is preferred.

The length of immobilization is case dependent and must be guided by clinical tenderness and pain on weight bearing. All symptoms must be resolved before any return to activity is allowed. Unexpected persistent symptoms should lead the physician to suspect patient noncompliance or a missed diagnosis.

Return to activity should be gentle and monitored closely. Dancers are generally good at knowing how to rehabilitate injuries; however, most have a tendency to advance too quickly.

STRESS FRACTURES

Stress fractures are spontaneous fractures that are the result of low-level repetitive stresses. These stresses in isolation are otherwise harmless [2] and often result in repetitive loading in bones subjected to continued episodes of low-level stress. They can occur in virtually every bone of the foot, lower leg, and ankle in dancers [3,4] and must be diagnosed in the early stages to avoid complete fracture.

Fibular Stress Fractures

A common stress fracture in the dance population is that of the fibula. Tenderness directly on the fibula shaft should precipitate a high index of suspicion for a fibular stress fracture. It is most often seen in the distal aspect of the fibula, commonly occurring in the distal third of the shaft, approximately 10 cm above the lateral malleolus [5,6]. In dancers, these stress fractures are frequently the cause of poor balance and fatigue when initiating a turn. They most often occur in the weight-bearing leg or the ankle of support. The fracture may recur in the same area within months if training is resumed too quickly [6]. Radiographs are frequently negative, and bone scan may be justified when clinical suspicion exists. Epiphyseal fractures of the distal fibula must be considered in the skeletally immature dancer.

Cam boot immobilization and rest are usually sufficient for adequate healing to occur. These measures usually have a good prognosis, but return to full use and motion equal to that of the other foot may take up to 1 year [6].

Calcaneal Stress Fracture

These injuries often seem similar to plantar fascitis initially, with pain presenting in the plantar aspect of the heel with the first step in the morning or pain during the day when initiating walking. There is often tenderness along the medial and lateral wall of the calcaneus and along the plantar aspect of the tuberosity. Physical examination can demonstrate swelling and warmth over the calcaneus, but this is not an absolute requirement. Plain radiographs are often unremarkable (Fig. 1). Advanced imaging studies such as bone scan or MRI are generally required to diagnose a calcaneal stress fracture. Common treatment includes non-weight-bearing cast immobilization for a minimum of 4 to 8 weeks, but persistent symptoms usually result in longer periods in the boot [5].

Navicular Stress Fracture

Tarsal navicular stress fractures are relatively uncommon but can be the explanation for otherwise unexplainable midfoot pain. They often result from impact activities and lead to swelling and discomfort in the dorsomedial aspect of the foot or arch. Areas of increased warmth and edema are frequently found in this region, and these must be differentiated from posterior tibial tendonitis. MRI shows bone marrow edema in the absence of posterior tibial tenosynovitis. Sometimes increased or decreased density of the bone is apparent along the area of affected navicular. In more advanced injuries, the fracture line (Fig. 2) may be surrounded by sclerotic bone and may split the navicular from the

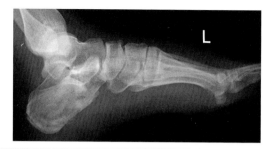

Fig. 1. Lateral radiograph of the foot demonstrating an acute calcaneal fracture. Although this injury was secondary to significant non-dance-related trauma, it was thought that an existing stress injury was contributory.

talonavicular joint to the naviculocuneiform joint. Chronic cases often exhibit sclerosis and fragmentation of the navicular dorsally, which can be a career-threatening injury in the professional dancer [5]. Conservative treatment most often includes 6 to 8 weeks in a non-weight-bearing cast [4]. A bone stimulator device may prove useful in difficult cases.

From a surgical perspective, there are two types of navicular fractures. Sagittal plane fractures are the most typical navicular stress fracture. Surgical treatment is often recommended, and it is usually 6 to 12 weeks before resumption of full dance activities can occur. The second injury type concerns the os navicular, which can present with pain prominence and edema at the medial navicular.

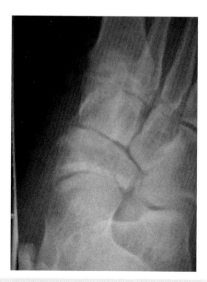

Fig. 2. Oblique radiograph of the foot demonstrating a fracture line in the sagittal plane of the navicular, with extension into the talonavicular joint.

There are several approaches for treating the os navicular and the tearing of the synostosis between the os navicular. One option is to excise the os navicular and advance or re-establish proper tension between the tendon and the main navicular. Alternately, the junction between the os navicular and the main navicular can be exposed, resecting the synostosis, establishing healthy bleeding surfaces, and reattaching the os navicular to the main navicular with one or two screws [5]. The decision to proceed with surgery should be given great consideration because full recovery takes many months and return to full dance activity can be difficult. Nakayama and colleagues [7] demonstrated an 80% bony union rate with perforation of the accessory navicular with several passes of a 1.0-mm K-wire in patients who had a skeletally immature first proximal phalanx.

Second Metatarsal Stress Fracture

The most common stress fracture site in dancers is that of the second metatarsal. It is the longest metatarsal and thus bears the bulk of the weight in the demipointe position. As a result, diaphyseal cortical thickening may often be seen on the dancer's radiograph. This role of increased weight bearing frequently leads to fatigue fractures [8]. Stress fractures at the base of the second metatarsal (Fig. 3) cause midfoot pain. Tenderness and warmth over the base of the second metatarsal are common but can also be due to synovitis of the second metatarsocuneiform joint from overloading during en pointe or demipointe. These injuries can be difficult to differentiate from synovitis of the Lisfranc's joint; both have activity-related pain and local tenderness [4]. It is frequently

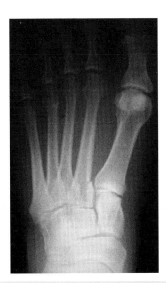

Fig. 3. Anteroposterior radiograph of the foot demonstrating a fracture of the base of the second metatarsal.

necessary to use MRI to properly diagnose the injury. Treatment often necessitates relative rest and avoidance of the offending activity for a 6- to 8-week period [5].

Kadel and colleagues [8] reported second metatarsal stress fractures in 63% of dancers. Controversy exists as to whether relative second metatarsal length factors into causality of second metatarsal stress fractures. Davidson and colleagues [9] found no variance in second metatarsal length or second toe length between dancers diagnosed with a second metatarsal stress fracture and dancers who did not have evidence of second metatarsal injury.

FIFTH METATARSAL FRACTURES

Fracture of the fifth metatarsal often results from inversion-related fatigue. Tired lateral calf muscles and peroneals lead to a loss of fine coordination through muscle fatigue, which causes injury. Choreography can also be blamed because certain sequences can place the dancer in a susceptible position to injury. There are many subtypes of fifth metatarsal fracture.

Stress fractures of the proximal fifth metatarsal diaphysis are usually due to repetitive adduction forces such as cutting or pivoting and are more frequently seen in modern dancers. They present with a low level of chronic lateral foot pain. Radiographs can demonstrate cortical thickening, periosteal reaction, and possibly a fracture line surrounded by sclerosis in chronic presentations. These cases usually require operative internal fixation with possible bone grafting because they have a high rate of nonunion with closed treatment methods [1]. In more subtle cases, peroneus brevis tendonitis at the insertion of the tuberosity is often difficult to distinguish from a periosteal stress reaction or subacute stress fracture.

Tuberosity fractures are often the result of missed jump landings and rolling over the outer border of the foot while in demipointe. Pain presents laterally, with tenderness, swelling, and ecchymosis. Avulsion fractures of the proximal fifth metatarsal are often associated with inversion injury and lateral ankle sprains. The fracture line is through the tuberosity and is usually extra-articular. Debate exists about the etiology of this injury because the long plantar ligament and peroneus brevis attach near this location. Dancers can usually bear weight but do so with pain. Treatment depends on the location of the fracture and is usually determined by symptomatology. A stiff-soled shoe or a removable cast boot is generally employed. Even if displaced, tuberosity fractures usually only require symptomatic treatment, and resumption to full activity can occur from 2 to 12 weeks. Occasionally these injuries progress to nonunion. Surgery may be necessary for these isolated cases [5].

Oblique spiral shaft fractures (Fig. 4), commonly known as "dancer's fracture" [10] are typically extra-articular. They start in the distal-lateral direction and run proximal-medially. Most commonly, a dancer rolls over the outer border of the foot while in demipointe position on the ball of the foot, with the ankle fully plantar flexed. Prior injury has a great impact on recurrence of this injury; in one study, 8 of the 35 dancers who had this injury reported

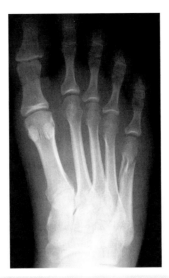

Fig. 4. Anteroposterior radiograph of the foot demonstrating a spiral fracture of the distal fifth metatarsal shaft.

a history of ankle instability before this injury. Pain and swelling in the lateral forefoot is common. The amount of displacement depends on the energy of the causal twisting injury, landing, or axial loading of the foot in the supinated position [5]. A limited open reduction is sometimes indicated in the higher-energy injuries, particularly when the dancer performs at an elite level.

Jones fractures (Fig. 5) occur at the metaphyseal–diaphyseal junction of the fifth metatarsal, with extension to the medial side of the metatarsal at the fourth or fifth metatarsal articulation [4]. These fractures, which are most common in modern dancers, are transverse and demonstrate a predilection for nonunion because of poor blood supply. As a result, many dancers show prolonged healing times with closed treatment, and high-level dancers, in particular, often choose surgery to avoid prolonged immobilization [1].

SESAMOIDS

The sesamoids lie in the tendons of the flexor hallucis brevis and articulate with the facets of the plantar surface of the first metatarsal just proximal to the metatarsophalangeal (MTP) joint. They bear weight during gait and increase the mechanical advantage of the flexor hallucis brevis, and are thus subject to considerable force in dance. This force can particularly be seen with rolling through the foot into demipointe or full pointe. In addition, the medial sesamoid bears more stress as dancers walk toed-out, thus forcing the line of progression to exit the foot medially under the first MTP joint rather than moving laterally between the first and second toes.

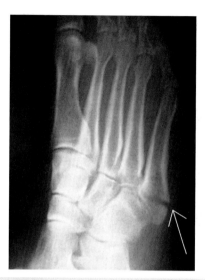

Fig. 5. Oblique radiograph of the foot demonstrating a Jones-type fracture of the fifth metatarsal (*arrow*).

The sesamoids are susceptible to numerous injuries, including inflammation, contusion, acute or stress fracture, osteonecrosis, and osteoarthritis. Pain localizes in the vicinity of the plantar surface of the first MTP joint. There is often tenderness over the sesamoid, with the medial tibial more commonly involved than the lateral. Pain may be provoked by resisted MTP flexion, and passive dorsiflexion may be painful, restricted, or both. Treatment is usually symptomatic, with immobilization and placement of a donut-shaped felt pad (0.375-in thick) beneath the tender area of the sesamoid for relief. Recovery may require a prolonged time away from dance [6]. Technical errors cause excessive loading and must be addressed. Improper landing also exacerbates the injury.

The bursa under the sesamoids can also become swollen and inflamed, resulting in bursitis. Palpation of the swollen bursa is often a subtle but important distinction. Local diagnostic injection of a limited amount of lidocaine (0.3 mL) can be helpful. Bipartite sesamoids are common, but their rounded edges seen on radiographs can help distinguish them from the sharply defined edges of an acute sesamoid fracture.

Sesamoiditis occurs in dancers who routinely engage in activities requiring the slapping of the forefoot and who perform frequent leaps. Initially the ball of the foot becomes tender, and within as short a period as 1 month, the area beneath the medial sesamoid becomes painful. The result is often a compression fracture of the tibiofibular sesamoid. Bone scans, CT, and MRI (Fig. 6) are necessary to differentiate these diagnoses.

Fracture of the sesamoid occurs from landing after a leap and is most commonly encountered in the tibial sesamoid. This injury can cause prolonged

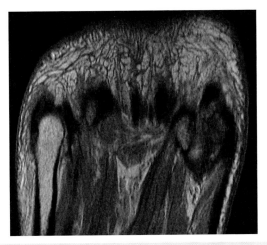

Fig. 6. Axial MRI demonstrating a fracture in the medial tibial sesamoid.

disability in dancers. Excision of chronically symptomatic sesamoids should be considered with great caution, particularly in the dancer.

PHALANGEAL FRACTURES

Phalangeal fatigue fractures occur but are rare. The injured toe can be taped to the adjacent, noninjured toes, with placement of a cotton pad in the web space for 3 weeks. The toe of the ballet or pointe shoe should be padded with lamb's wool to relieve pressure [6].

Acute strain of the interphalangeal joint of the hallux is sometimes seen in ballet students using pointe shoes lacking sufficient stiffness in the toe box. Initially there is en pointe pain and swelling and an inability to dance sur les pointes. Diagnosis can be made by a gentle rotation of the distal phalanx of the hallux while holding the MTP joint, which causes pain over the dorsum and sides of the joint.

Chronic hyperflexion of the interphalangeal joint of the hallux is sometimes apparent in children. This condition results from allowing students to dance en pointe before their ability, training, balance, and maturity dictate [6].

DISLOCATION OF TOES

Strain of the MTP joints of the lateral toes is common (occasionally occurring during accidents such as striking one's foot against the scenery) and can cause the dislocation of the proximal interphalangeal or MTP joint, which is immediately incapacitating. Dorsal displacement of the phalanx causes obvious deformity. Treatment includes closed reduction by hyperextending the joint and applying traction to pull the phalanx distally and then flexing the toe to reduce the deformity. Subsequently the toe needs to be taped to the adjacent uninjured toe for approximately 3 weeks [6].

SUMMARY

Fractures in the dance population are common. A high index of suspicion should be considered for a stress fracture due to the repetitive nature of dance and the prevalence of poor nutrition in the dancer. Radiography, CT, MRI, and bone scan should be used as necessary to arrive at the correct diagnosis after meticulous physical examination. Treatment should address the fracture itself and any surrounding problems such as nutritional/hormonal issues and training/performance techniques and regimens. Compliance issues in this population are a concern, so treatment strategies should be tailored accordingly. Stress fractures in particular can present difficulties to the treating physician and may require prolonged treatment periods.

References

[1] Kadel NJ. Foot and ankle injuries in dance. Phys Med Rehabil Clin N Am 2006;17(4): 813–26.

[2] Muscolo L, Migues A, Slullitel G, et al. Stress fracture nonunion at the base of the second metatarsal in a ballet dancer: a case report. Am J Sports Med 2004;32(6):1535–7.

[3] Hillier JC, Peace K, Hulme A, et al. Pictoral review: MRI features of foot and ankle injuries in ballet dancers. Br J Radiol 2004;77(918):532–7.

[4] Macintyre J, Joy E. Foot and ankle injuries in dance. Clin Sports Med 2000;19(2):351–68.

[5] Myerson MS. Foot and ankle disorders. vol. 2. Philadelphia: WB Saunders Company; 2000. p. 1462.

[6] Jahss MH. Disorders of the foot and ankle. 2nd edition. Philadelphia: WB Saunders Company; 1991. p. 3491.

[7] Nakayama S, Sugimoto K, Takakura Y, et al. Percutaneous drilling of symptomatic accessory navicular in young athletes. Am J Sports Med 2005;33(4):531–5.

[8] Kadel NJ, Teitz CC, Kronmal RA. Stress fractures in ballet dancers. Am J Sports Med 1992;20(4):445–9.

[9] Davidson G, Pizzari T, Mayes S. The influence of second toe and metatarsal length on stress fractures at the base of the second metatarsal in classical dancers. Foot Ankle Int 2007;28(10):1082–6.

[10] O'Malley MJ, Hamilton WG, Munyak J. Fractures of the distal shaft of the fifth metatarsal. 'Dancer's fracture.' Am J Sports Med 1996;24(2):240–3.

Clin Sports Med 27 (2008) 305–320

ELSEVIER
SAUNDERS

CLINICS IN SPORTS MEDICINE

Forefoot Injuries in Dancers

Victor R. Prisk, MD, Padhraig F. O'Loughlin, MD,
John G. Kennedy, MD, MMSc, MCh, FRCSI, FRCS (Orth)*

Foot and Ankle Department, Hospital for Special Surgery, 523 East 72nd Street,
Suite 514, New York, NY 10021, USA

D ancers, particularly ballet dancers, are artists and athletes. In dance, the choreographer acts as a sculptor, using the dancer as a medium of expression. This often entails placing the dancer's body in positions that require extraordinary flexibility and movement, which requires controlled power and endurance. Ballet and other forms of dance can be highly demanding activities, with a lifetime injury incidence of up to 90% [1]. Ballet is stressful particularly on the dancer's forefoot. The en pointe position of maximal plantarflexion through the forefoot, midfoot, and hindfoot requires tremendous flexibility and strength that only can be attained safely through many years of training. The forces experienced by the toes and metatarsals are extraordinary.

Injuries to the forefoot can occur as a result of acute trauma, such as during a leap or as a result of stress caused by repetitive micro-trauma that is dependent upon training volume and intensity. Acute trauma can occur because of central fatigue, muscle weakness, equipment malfunction, or inappropriate progression of skill attainment. The dancer and the choreographer need to be aware of over-training and the dancer's physiologic well being. Also, they must recognize that injury may occur with rapid increases in training volume, which leads to stress on bones, ligaments, and tendons that are not conditioned to accept the load. These injuries may cause the dancer to accommodate by altering learned dance technique and by subjecting themselves to abnormal stresses on the rest of the foot, ankle, and kinetic chain.

In addition to training volume, dancers must recognize the importance of proper nutrition and general health to prevent injury. In particular, female dancers may experience the "female athlete triad" of disordered eating, menstrual irregularities, and osteopenia [2]. Deficiencies of growth hormone, IGF-1, and estrogen may contribute to a delay in healing of fractures and chronic injuries [3,4]. Similarly, decreased availability of calcium and vitamin D with subsequent secondary hyperparathyroidism may contribute to osteopenia and subsequent delayed unions or stress fractures [5].

*Corresponding author. E-mail address: kennedyj@hss.edu (J.G. Kennedy).

0278-5919/08/$ – see front matter
doi:10.1016/j.csm.2007.12.005

This article focuses on injuries acquired acutely or by chronic stress to the forefoot. Dance presents the physician with common and unique problems to the forefoot. The authors explore injuries to the great toe, lesser toes, and metatarsals.

THE GREAT TOE
Toenails
Dancers' toenails take a beating, especially in ballet technique shoes en pointe. Modified ballet shoes more evenly distribute pressure away from the toes, but total force cannot be reduced [6]. Acute injuries to the toenails include avulsions or subungual hematomas. An avulsion should be treated with meticulous wound care and should concentrate on preventing closure of the germinal matrix by interposition of the avulsed nail. Any lacerations to the sterile matrix should be repaired and the nail should be left in place to be pushed off the nail bed by the regenerating nail. Painful subungual hematomas should be drained using a battery operated electrocautery. These hematomas may be recurrent and cause chronic pain in the dancer, causing loss of time in rehearsal or on stage. Rarely, subungual hematoma may necessitate nail excision. It is recommended that dancers regularly monitor their nails and avoid wearing polish, so they can detect any early signs of hematoma.

Most infections of the toenails are either bacterial or fungal. Acute paronychia often is caused by a bacterial infection. Treatment may require drainage while patients are under local anesthesia and on antibiotics. A chronic paronychia is often the result of fungal infection. Brittle, thick, discolored nails may indicate a fungal infection (onychomycosis). If problematic, this may be treated with oral antifungal agents that require regular surveillance of liver function tests, which are expensive. Alternative topical treatments (urea, oils, antifungals, and so forth) also may be effective. In a study at the University of Rochester, 100% tea tree oil applied twice daily in conjunction with debridement improved nail appearance and symptomatology similar to treatment with topical 1% clotrimazole and debridement [7]. Likewise, onychocryptosis, or ingrown toenails, can result in severe pain and infection. These can be treated initially by warm saline soaks and antibiotics if an infection is suspected. One should not attempt to trim the corner of the nail, because this action could make the condition worse. This causes the nail to form a fish hook deformity that grows further into the nail groove. Surgical treatment may be required and consists of wedge resection at the nail groove, phenolization of the nail matrix, or partial matricectomy and nail removal.

Inspection of the nails can provide information about the internal working of the body as well. Splitting and fraying of the nails are associated with deficiencies of folic acid, vitamin C, and protein. Also, spooning, flattening, or grooves forming in the nails may indicate iron or vitamin B12 deficiency. Muehrcke's lines are white lines crossing the nails often associated with hypoalbuminemia. These findings are of particular importance in caring for the dancer who may be at risk for eating disorders and resultant malnutrition.

Phalanges and Interphalangeal Joint

Weight bearing activities, such as running and performing jumps or leaps, result in ground reaction forces several times greater than that of bodyweight at the phalanges. These forces combined with classical ballet training practices, increases in training volume, eating disorders, secondary amenorrhea, and osteopenia can result in phalangeal stress fractures. These have been documented to occur in female athletes at the distal and proximal phalanx [8,9]. Hallux valgus may be a predisposing risk factor for an avulsion-type stress fracture of the proximal phalanx [8]. Tensile strain on the medial collateral ligament and insertion of the medial head of the flexor hallucis brevis may lead to an avulsion-type stress fracture of the medial base of the proximal phalanx.

Nussbaum and colleagues [10] demonstrated that bone scintigraphy can be used to detect stress reactions and stress fractures in both asymptomatic and symptomatic sites in the ballet dancer. MRI also can be used to differentiate traumatic synovitis from stress reactions in ballet dancers [9,11]. The physician must keep a high index of suspicion for these fractures. Conservative treatment with a short period of nonweightbearing (2–3 weeks) and gradual return to activities should manage these stress fractures. Attention should be paid to training volume, nutrition, and the general health of the dancer during this time. If the dancer has continuous pain, follow-up studies should be performed to rule out the possibility of nonunion. Surgical excision of the nonunion with cancellous calcaneal bone graft and screw fixation may be warranted.

In young dancers, hyperflexion injuries of the interphalangeal joint (IPJ) can occur when attempting to go en pointe. Here, weight is distributed over the nail and dorsum of the toe in the pointe shoe. Hyperextension of the IPJ also can occur, often to compensate for lack of motion in the metatarsophalangeal (MTP) joint. This rarely needs surgical intervention despite radiographic appearances, because the joint is quite accommodating and typically asymptomatic. In patients who do complain of symptoms, lambs wool wrapping can help alleviate the discomfort. Hallux valgus interphalangeus, or adduction of the distal phalanx, can occur because of traumatic disruption of the collateral ligaments, intra-articular fractures of the proximal phalanx, or acquired deformity at the interphalangeal joint. Radiographs are essential to evaluate the origin of this deformity. In some instances, surgical repair may be required. The alternative, fusion of the IPJ in a dancer, is discouraged.

First Metatarsophalangeal Joint

Hallux valgus

It was believed widely at one time that dancing played a role in the pathogenesis of hallux valgus (Fig. 1). However, a study of active and retired ballet dancers in Stockholm, Sweden showed no increase in the valgus angulation of the hallux compared with that of non-dancers [12]. Conversely, more recent evidence showed a statistically significant increase in hallux valgus deformity in ballet dancers [13]. Dancers, like the rest of the population, may be resistant or prone to develop hallux valgus, which may have a familial inheritance [14]. In those

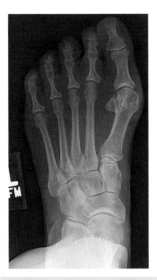

Fig. 1. X-ray depicting hallux valgus in a modern dancer.

dancers that are prone to develop hallux valgus, it is imperative to delay surgical intervention for as long as possible. Dance en pointe and demi-pointe requires extremes of plantarflexion and dorsiflexion of the first MTP joint, respectively. Hallux valgus surgery often adversely affects this critical motion of the MTP joint. Jones and colleagues [15] elegantly demonstrated loss of first MTP joint dorsiflexion with distal soft tissue release and proximal metatarsal osteotomy in a cadaveric model. Thus, well-meaning bunion surgery inadvertently can end a dancer's career. Most cases of hallux valgus can be treated conservatively with toe spacers and horseshoe pads. If a conservatively treated bunion is precluding a dancer from activity and surgical intervention is warranted, then one may consider a chevron osteotomy with isometric capsular repair to avoid compromised motion.

Hallux rigidus

The dancer needs 90° to 100° of first MTP joint dorsiflexion for proper dance technique [16]. Any restriction of this first MTP joint motion will prevent the dancer from performing releve or demi-pointe, where the dancer stands on the ball of the foot. The dancer may actively or inadvertently accommodate for this by supinating the foot to off-load the great toe. This rolling onto the lateral border of the foot is known in dance as "sickling" and affects the kinetic chain proximally. The varus moment from the forefoot may increase the risk of inversion injuries at the ankle and fractures of the fifth metatarsal. Hallux rigidus is a spectrum of first MTP joint degenerative arthritis that results in a restriction of joint motion, primarily in dorsiflexion (Fig. 2). The symptoms result from cartilage wear, altered joint mechanics, and osteophyte formation, particularly on the dorsal aspect of the first metatarsal head. Hallux rigidus usually

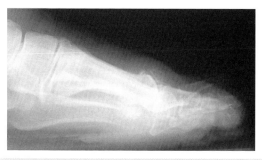

Fig. 2. X-ray depicting hallux rigidus with characteristic loss of joint space.

causes pain from joint impingement of dorsal osteophytes, joint inflammation or synovitis, and shoe-related pressure on prominent osteophytes. Pain during range-of-motion also may be related to the irregularity of the articular cartilage surface and varying degress of cartilage erosion.

Hallux rigidus likely results from repetitive microtrauma to the first MTP joint cartilage or may result from a single traumatic event. Traumatic events can result in an osteochondral defect in the first metatarsal head. There are case reports of autogenous osteochondral graft transfer for first metatarsal osteochondral defects with functional return of joint motion [17]. However, this needs to be studied with regards to range of motion required to dance. Further treatment of hallux rigidus and first MTP joint arthritis depends on the grade of disease. In 1988, Hattrup and Johnson [18] described a radiographic grading system for hallux rigidus as follows:

Grade 1: Joint space maintained with minimal spurring and mild degeneration
Grade 2: Joint-space narrowing, with bony proliferation on the metatarsal head and phalanx and subchondral sclerosis or cysts
Grade 3: Severe joint-space narrowing, extensive bony proliferation, loose bodies or a dorsal ossicle.

Coughlin and Shurnas [19] proposed a classification system based on range of motion in addition to radiographic and examination findings as follows:

Grade 0: Normal radiograph, no pain, only stiffness or slight loss of MTP joint motion
Grade 1: Intermittent joint pain, mild restriction of motion, minor narrowing of joint space on radiographs
Grade 2: More constant joint pain, moderate restriction of motion, moderate joint space narrowing with osteophyte formation
Grade 3: Constant joint pain, no pain at midrange motion, less than 20° of total motion (moderately severe restriction), extensive osteophytes and severe joint space narrowing
Grade 4 : Same as grade 3, but on examination, patient exhibits midrange pain on passive manipulation of the MTP joint.

Treatment for grades 0 to 1 hallux rigidus is mainly conservative. Physical therapy and modalities may help improve range of motion and limit pain. The physician may consider joint injections with either cortisone or viscosupplementation. For grade 2 disease that has failed conservative management, cheilectomy with resection of marginal osteophytes may we warranted. Up to one third of the dorsal metatarsal head may be resected [20]. A dorsal based closing wedge Moberg osteotomy of the proximal phalanx may improve dorsiflexion at the expense of plantarflexion. This loss of plantarflexion needs to be discussed with the dancer preoperatively.

Intraoperative dorsiflexion often overestimates the motion that can be expected following surgery. Up to half of what is achieved intraoperatively will be evident at follow-up examination. It is important for dancers to have realistic expectations of surgery. Although surgery can reduce pain and symptoms, a dancer's joint will never be normal. Also, there may be a long recovery time, with full recovery taking up to 6 months.

There are no great options for grade 3 hallux rigidus in dancers. This may be treated with cheilectomy and cartilage restoration procedures, such as microfracture, osteochondral autograft transfer, or interpositional arthroplasty (Figs. 3 and 4). To avoid the career ending arthrodesis in grade 3 and 4 disease, interpositional arthroplasty can be performed with reproducible outcomes [21]. It is important to select these patients carefully and avoid over-shortening of the proximal phalanx (25% to 30% at most). A foreshortened first ray in these patients may cause transfer metatarsalgia and an increased risk of second metatarsal stress reactions.

Sesamoid injuries

The hallucal sesamoid bones lie within the substance of the flexor hallucis brevis tendons and bear up to 50% of bodyweight. They may experience forces greater than three times bodyweight during leaps and toe push-off during dance. The sesamoids increase the mechanical advantage of the flexor hallucis brevis, assist with weightbearing under the first metatarsal, and elevate the first metatarsal head off the ground. The hallucal sesamoids may be bipartite in up to 25% of patients (affecting the tibial sesamoid more frequently) and may be bilateral in up to 85%.

The sesamoids commonly are injured in dancers either acutely or because of repetitive stress. Acute injury can occur in those who fail to perform a plie on landing, which absorbs the energy of the floor by landing through partially flexed knees. Without the absorption built into the dancer's technique, sudden deceleration with high impact of the sesamoid bones predisposes to injury. Pirouettes in demi-pointe stance combined with a "model's foot" (which has a long first ray with an exaggerated cascade from the first to fifth) ray results in extra stress to the sesamoids.

The differential diagnosis of sesamoid pain is lengthy and requires a careful history and physical examination. A history and physical examination

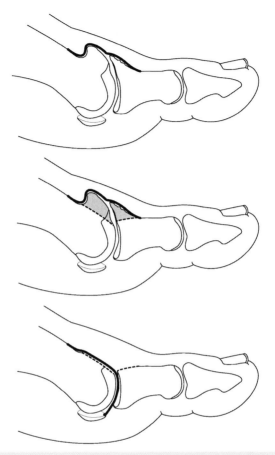

Fig. 3. Sequential drawings illustrating interpositional arthroplasty procedure. Capsule of first metatarsophalangeal joint is interposed between the head of the first metatarsal and the base of the proximal phalanx of the hallux.

combined with x-rays, MRI, or CT scan aids in the diagnosis. The differential diagnosis may include:

- Sesamoiditis
- Stess fracture of the sesamoid bone (Fig. 5)
- Avulsion fracture or sprain of the sesamoid complex
- Sprain of a bipartite sesamoid with widening between two fragments
- Arthrosis of the sesamoid-metatarsal articulation
- Osteonecrosis of the sesamoid.

Sesamoiditis is a painful inflammation of the region surrounding the sesamoid apparatus that is caused by repetitive, excessive pressure on the ball of the foot. Most of the time, sesamoiditis can be treated with a felt pad around

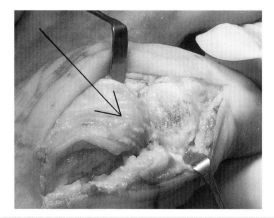

Fig. 4. Intraoperative image of capsule interposed between distal first metatarsal and proximal phalanx of the great toe.

the sesamoid ("dancer's pad") to distribute forces and offload the painful sesamoid. In general, symptoms will resolve without additional interventions, but this may take up to 6 months and modification of training volume for complete resolution. If further diagnostic testing is required, an MRI can be helpful. In patients wjo have recalcitrant pain for more than 6 months after initial treatment, surgery is warranted. A medial incision can be used for tibial sesamoidectomy, whereas a plantar or dorsal first web space incision is needed for fibular sesamoidectomy. A partial excision based on MRI findings is preferred to prevent varus or valgus malalignment of the great toe.

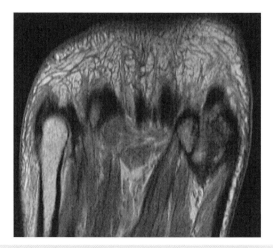

Fig. 5. MRI showing a fracture of the medial sesamoid.

Sesamoid bursitis, sesamoid instability, and nerve entrapment are all conditions that may mimic sesamoiditis but have distinct treatments as follows:

- Sesamoid bursitis. Inflammation and swelling of the bursa is often misdiagnosed as sesamoiditis. However, careful physical examination usually can identify a symptomatic swollen bursa when present. The bursa can be palpated and injected with corticosteroid and local anesthetic for treatment. The addition of a dancer's pad can resolve the problem without surgery. This condition often takes time to resolve and may be complicated by fibrous scar tissue that can be painful and restrict motion later. These rubbing bands of scar tissue can be excised with a bursectomy through a plantar medial incision. Care must be taken to identify and protect the proper digital nerve during the approach, and meticulous skin closure is critical for a good outcome.
- Sesamoid instability. In the rare instance that the medial collateral ligament of the tibial sesamoid may be torn, the sesamoid dislocates laterally in releve. On barefoot examination, a sudden clunk occurs when the sesamoids slip laterally into the first webspace. This condition requires surgical repair, much like recurrent patella dislocations. The medial ligamentous structures are reconstructed at the isometric center of motion to avoid overtightening the MTP joint. The reconstructed ligament is anchored through a metatarsal head, pull-through stitch, or suture anchor. Rehabilitation includes early joint motion and a toe spacer to protect the repair.
- Nerve entrapment. Either the medial plantar nerve (Joplin's neuroma) or lateral plantar nerve to the hallux can become entrapped under the tibial or fibular sesamoid, respectively. The condition causes neuropathic symptoms and a positive Tinel's sign. Symptoms may be relieved with local anesthetic, and this may be diagnostic. Medial entrapment tends to occur in dancers who pronate. Treatment for chronic cases of medial entrapment may include neurolysis, nerve transposition, or neurectomy. Lateral entrapment is more difficult to diagnose by Tinel's sign, thus the diagnostic injection into the area of the nerve as it exits from beneath the deep transverse ligament insertion into the fibular sesamoid is more useful. If symptoms are disabling, surgical release of the deep transverse ligament often relieves nerve compression.

THE LESSER TOES
Metatarsophalangeal Joints
Freiberg's infarction
Freiberg's infarction may be more common in women, but it is not more common in dancers than in the general population. This disease of the lesser metatarsal heads more often affects the second metatarsal (Fig. 6). Freiberg's infarction presents as metatarsalgia and MTP joint pain and swelling. In general, radiographs lag behind clinical symptoms by up to 6 months. Bone scan or MRI facilitates an earlier diagnosis. The following four types of infraction occur:

- Type I: Localized osteonecrosis of the metatarsal head healing by creeping substitution. The head heals completely with little or no defect.
- Type II: Osteonecrosis results in collapse of the dorsal portion of the metatarsal head during revascularization. A dorsal ridge and osteophytes form limiting dorsiflexion. Dorsal exostectomy often is curative, restoring motion.

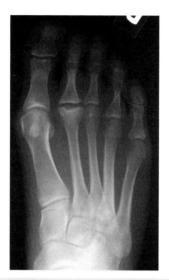

Fig. 6. X-ray showing Freiberg's disease of second metatarsal head with flattening of articular surface.

- Type III: The dorsal head collapses and the articular surface loosens and falls into the joint. Often, the plantar aspect of the joint is intact and can be left alone. However, simple dorsal exostectomy is not sufficient to restore the damaged joint, and a capsular arthroplasty is required [22].
- Type IV: This is a very rare entity in which several heads are involved. This may represent a congenital epiphyseal dysplasia rather than a true infraction. Each head must be treated individually.

Metatarsophalangeal joint instability

Metatarsalgia is not common in dancers. When it is encountered, physicians should suspect Freiberg's infarction or MTP joint instability. As the dancer goes en demi-pointe or in releve on the ball of the foot, the proximal phalanx subluxes dorsally, pushing the metatarsal head plantar-ward and causing pain. The demi-pointe position transmits excessive loads through the second and third MTP joints. Physical examination is critical, because this dynamic problem often can go unrecognized on x-ray. The dancer has plantar pain to palpation and dorsal pain when asked to releve. Examination also will reveal passive translation in the anterior-posterior plane, resulting in subluxation or dislocation of the MTP joint (Lachman test of the MTP joint) [22]. Treatment initially is conservative, with taping to adjacent toes or to the plantar surface with stress-relieving padding. Once the ligaments and plantar plate are over-stretched, the condition becomes chronic and necessitates surgery. Flexor to extensor transfers are not a good option for dancers because of an unacceptable amount of residual stiffness [23]. Correction includes a very limited resection arthroplasty with a plantar condylectomy or a limited Weil osteotomy. Resection relieves metatarsalgia by redistributing plantar surface pressure and allows for healing of the plantar plate through scarring to the resected plantar condyle. A toe wire should be used for 2 weeks, and early motion can be started thereafter.

Dislocation of the metatarsophalangeal joints
Acute injuries, more common in males because of a lack of protective toe box, should be reduced and immobilized until soft-tissue healing can occur. These injuries may go undiagnosed, because they are disguised by toe swelling. In such instances of chronic dislocation, a limited resection arthroplasty or Weil osteotomy may facilitate reduction.

Idiopathic metatarsophalangeal synovitis
Synovitis resulting in a swollen "sausage-like" toe may cause joint laxity or result from joint laxity. It is more likely that chronic stress to the plantar plate in dancers results in joint laxity and irritation of the joint. The inflammation can be controlled with anti-inflammatory medication and taping. When the condition is resistant to conservative management, surgical exploration is required. Again, surgical treatment addresses the instability with limited resection arthroplasty with plantar condylectomy or Weil osteotomy if the affected ray is long or plantarflexed.

Miscellaneous Lesser Toe Problems

Unstable fifth proximal interphalangeal joint
An untreated lateral dislocation of the fifth proximal interphalangeal (PIP) joint with rupture of the medial collateral ligament may become a chronically unstable joint. The patient may notice only pain or may even mention that the toe dislocates. Applying a valgus force to the toe elicits pain or dislocation that the dancer recognizes as the problem when dancing. Buddy tapping the toe to the fourth toe usually helps. If surgery is needed, a PIP resection with placement of a K-wire results in stabilizing scar tissue formation. The K-wire is removed in 2–3 weeks, and buddy tapping is applied again.

Bunionette
Similar to hallux valgus of the first ray, a bunionette is a varus deviation of the fifth toe that presents as pain with shoe wear (Fig. 7). Physiologically, the 4-5 intermetatarsal angle and fifth MTP joint angle average 6.2° and 10.2° respectively [24,25]. Patients who have an increased 4–5 intermetatarsal angle tend to be more symptomatic. Three types of bunionettes are described below:

- Type I: Simple enlargement of fifth metatarsal head with lateral prominence
- Type II: Congenital lateral bowing of the fifth metatarsal shaft with symptomatic increase in the fifth MTP joint angle
- Type III: Increased 4–5 intermetatarsal angle with symptomatic increase in the fifth MTP joint angle.

Treatment typically is conservative, with shaving of hypertrophic callus and padding of the fifth metatarsal head. Painful lateral and plantar keratoses may

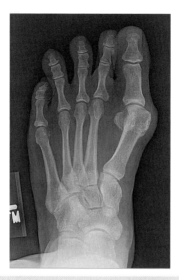

Fig. 7. Bunionette over fifth metatarsophalangeal joint. Patient has coexisting hallux valgus.

necessitate surgical intervention. Because of high recurrence of deformity and long recovery times, surgery often is postponed until retirement. Surgery may include simple lateral condylectomy for type I or a metatarsal osteotomy for type II or type III bunionettes. However, meticulous repair of the joint capsule and abductor digiti quinti muscle must be performed to limit the high recurrence of deformity and later dislocation of the MTP joint.

Mallet toe

A mallet toe is defined by a neutral MTP joint and PIP joint position with Distal Interphalangeal (DIP) joint flexion. Acute or chronic trauma to the DIP joint or extensor mechanism may result in a mallet toe, as when dancing en pointe. If pain and skin breakdown warrants surgery, a DIP resection with placement of a K-wire corrects the deformity. It often is unnecessary to tenotomize the long flexor tendon.

Corns, calluses, and blisters

Ballet dancers are very familiar with corns and calluses. This tough skin literally allows the dancer to tolerate and perform in pointe toe shoes. They may need occasional trimming or padding. Infection can occur under a corn and these should be unroofed and treated with antibiotics and magnesium sulfate soaks. In barefoot dance, large calluses may form with crevices that crack, resulting in possible sites for infection. Likewise, blisters, very common in dance of all types, may need to be unroofed and can be a nidus for infection. The dancer needs to watch for signs of local cellulitis, which should be treated with antibiotics and soaks.

THE METATARSALS
Second Metatarsal Stress Fracture

The rigors of ballet select for the mild cavus foot because of the mechanical advantage of a rigid forefoot for dancing en pointe. Nonetheless, this results in high forefoot stresses on impact. Although Wolff's law dictates the cortical hypertrophy often seen in the metatarsals of dancers, repeated microtrauma combined with systemic physiologic stress exceeds the reparative capacity of bone. Over time, this results in painful stress reactions and stress fractures. In particular, because of its tight keystone position between the cuneiforms, the second metatarsal base acts as a stress riser for fractures at the proximal metaphysis.

Various studies have investigated risk factors for stress fractures at the base of the second metatarsal (Fig. 8). O'Malley and colleagues [26] suggested that beyond dancing en pointe, nutritional deficits, low estrogen levels, over-training, and floor hardness may contribute to stress fractures. Multiple studies have correlated Morton's foot (short first metatarsal compared with second metatarsal) to an increased risk of second metatarsal base stress fractures [11,26,27]. Others have found that a longer second metatarsal in female dancers also results in more daily foot pain and are related to hallux rigidus without increased risk of fracture [28].

Pain and tenderness in the proximal portion of the second metatarsal is a stress fracture in the dancer until proven otherwise. Unfortunately, it is difficult sometimes to differentiate Lis Franc joint synovitis from stress reactions at the base of the second metatarsal. Additionally, x-rays often are difficult to evaluate in dancers who have physiologic cortical hypertrophy, and x-ray

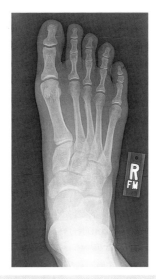

Fig. 8. Fracture of distal third metatarsal.

findings tend to lag behind symptoms. Harrington and colleagues [11] demonstrated that MRI can be useful in differentiating synovitis,and boney stress reactions and can aid in early diagnosis and treatment. Left untreated, the stress reactions progress to fractures with poorer outcomes.

These fractures require protection with a short-leg walking cast or cam walker boot if the dancer can be trusted. Fractures that are resistant to protected weightbearing and result in delayed-union can be managed further with ultrasound bone stimulators or surgery. It is important to address training volume and the female athlete triad. Expeditious referral to a nutritionist, endocrinologist, and sport psychologist is prudent if the female athlete triad is noted.

Dancer's Fracture of the Fifth Metatarsal

A spiral diaphyseal fracture of the distal fifth metatarsal is common in a dancer who rolls over the lateral border of the foot in demi pointe position [16,29]. The dancer who "sickles" in response to first MTP joint pain is at higher risk of this injury. Nonoperative care with protected weight-bearing for comfort is employed successfully with both nondisplaced fractures and significantly displaced fractures [29]. The relatively high mobility of the fifth metatarsal allows for malunion without great change in the mechanics of the forefoot. The long spiral nature of these fractures and thick periosteum produces predictable healing with pain free walking on average at 6 weeks and return to training and performance in 3 to 5 months.

SUMMARY

The dancer's forefoot takes a beating in training and performance. The physician, the dancer, the athletic trainer, and the dance master must work together to keep dancers healthy. Nearly all professional dancers employed for more than 1 year will have an injury, and the likelihood of that injury being in the foot or ankle is high [30]. Monitoring training volume and general health of the dancer helps to maximize the dancer's healing potential. Proper technique, sequential skill progression, and proper equipment useage may help limit acute injuries to the dancer's foot.

The orthopedist must pay close attention to the entire kinetic chain of the dancer. Injuries and chronic pain in the foot may precipitate additional injuries further up the kinetic chain as a compensatory response to the injury or because of inadequate rehabilitation. Apart from the history and physical examination, a biochemical and physiologic profile of the dancer should be obtained to discover and treat the female athlete triad. This will maximize healing potential. The orthopedist also must realize that the dancer often regards injury and pain as a way of life. They may have a fear of treatments that could result in loss of training time and possibly employment. The physician must be an advocate for the dancer who is an athlete and strive to provide an accurate diagnosis and an expeditious treatment strategy.

References

[1] Macintyre J, Joy E. Foot and ankle injuries in dance. Clin Sports Med 2000;19(2):351–68.

[2] Otis CL, Drinkwater B, Johnson M, et al. American College of Sports Medicine position stand. The Female Athlete Triad. Med Sci Sports Exerc 1997;29(5):1–9.

[3] Miller KK. Mechanisms by which nutritional disorders cause reduced bone mass in adults. J Womens Health 2003;12(2):145–50.

[4] Warren MP, Brooks-Gunn J, Fox RP, et al. Persistent osteopenia in ballet dancers with amenorrhea and delayed menarche despite hormone therapy: a longitudinal study. Fertil Steril 2003;80(2):398–404.

[5] Valimaki VV, Alfthan H, Lehmuskallio E, et al. Risk factors for clinical stress fractures in male military recruits: a prospective cohort study. Bone 2005;37(2):267–73.

[6] Miller CD, Paulos LE, Parker RD, et al. The ballet technique shoe: a preliminary study of eleven differently modified ballet technique shoes using force and pressure plates. Foot Ankle 1990;11(2):97–100.

[7] Buck DS, Nidorf DM, Addino JG. Comparison of two topical preparations for the treatment of onychomycosis: Melaleuca alternifolia (tea tree) oil and clotrimazole. J Fam Pract 1994;38(6):601–5.

[8] Pitsis GC, Best JP, Sullivan MR. Unusual stress fractures of the proximal phalanx of the great toe: a report of two cases. Br J Sports Med 2004;38(6):e31.

[9] Lo SL, Zoga AC, Elias I, et al. Stress fracture of the distal phalanx of the great toe in a professional ballet dancer: a case report. Am J Sports Med 2007;35(9):1564–6.

[10] Nussbaum AR, Treves ST, Micheli L. Bone stress lesions in ballet dancers: scintigraphic assessment. AJR Am J Roentgenol 1988;150(4):851–5.

[11] Harrington T, Crichton KJ, Anderson IF. Overuse ballet injury of the base of the second metatarsal. A diagnostic problem. Am J Sports Med 1993;21(4):591–8.

[12] Einarsdottir H, Troell S, Wykman A. Hallux valgus in ballet dancers: a myth? Foot Ankle Int 1995;16(2):92–4.

[13] van Dijk CN, Lim LS, Poortman A, et al. Degenerative joint disease in female ballet dancers. Am J Sports Med 1995;23(3):295–300.

[14] Pique-Vidal C, Sole MT, Antich J. Hallux valgus inheritance: pedigree research in 350 patients with bunion deformity. J Foot Ankle Surg 2007;46(3):149–54.

[15] Jones CP, Coughlin MJ, Grebing BR, et al. First metatarsophalangeal joint motion after hallux valgus correction: a cadaver study. Foot Ankle Int 2005;26(8):614–9.

[16] Hamilton WG. Foot and ankle injuries in dancers. Clin Sports Med 1988;7(1):143–73.

[17] Zelent ME, Neese DJ. Osteochondral autograft transfer of the first metatarsal head: a case report. J Foot Ankle Surg 2005;44(5):406–11.

[18] Hattrup SJ, Johnson KA. Subjective results of hallux rigidus following treatment with cheilectomy. Clin Orthop Relat Res 1988;226:182–91.

[19] Coughlin MJ, Shurnas PS. Hallux rigidus: demographics, etiology, and radiographic assessment. Foot Ankle Int 2003;24(10):731–43.

[20] Mann RA, Clanton TO. Hallux rigidus: treatment by cheilectomy. J Bone Joint Surg Am 1988;70(3):400–6.

[21] Hamilton WG, O'Malley MJ, Thompson FM, et al. Roger Mann Award 1995. Capsular interposition arthroplasty for severe hallux rigidus. Foot Ankle Int 1997;18(2):68–70.

[22] Thompson FM, Hamilton WG. Problems of the second metatarsophalangeal joint. Orthopedics 1987;10(1):83–9.

[23] Myerson MS, Jung HG. The role of toe flexor-to-extensor transfer in correcting metatarsophalangeal joint instability of the second toe. Foot Ankle Int 2005;26(9):675–9.

[24] Nestor BJ, Kitaoka HB, Ilstrup DM, et al. Radiologic anatomy of the painful bunionette. Foot Ankle 1990;11(1):6–11.

[25] Fallat LM, Buckholz J. An analysis of the tailor's bunion by radiographic and anatomical display. J Am Podiatry Assoc 1980;70(12):597–603.

[26] O'Malley MJ, Hamilton WG, Munyak J, et al. Stress fractures at the base of the second meta-tarsal in ballet dancers. Foot Ankle Int 1996;17(2):89–94.

[27] Chuckpaiwong B, Cook C, Pietrobon R, et al. Second metatarsal stress fracture in sport: comparative risk factors between proximal and non-proximal locations. Br J Sports Med 2007;41(8):510–4.

[28] Ogilvie-Harris DJ, Carr MM, Fleming PJ. The foot in ballet dancers: the importance of second toe length. Foot Ankle Int 1995;16(3):144–7.

[29] O'Malley MJ, Hamilton WG, Munyak J. Fractures of the distal shaft of the fifth metatarsal. "Dancer's fracture". Am J Sports Med 1996;24(2):240–3.

[30] Nilsson C, Leanderson J, Wykman A, et al. The injury panorama in a Swedish professional ballet company. Knee Surg Sports Traumatol Arthrosc 2001;9(4):242–6.

Clin Sports Med 27 (2008) 321–328

CLINICS IN SPORTS MEDICINE

ELSEVIER
SAUNDERS

Bunions in Dancers

John G. Kennedy, MD, MMSc, MCh, FRCSI, FRCS (Orth)[a,*],
Jean Allain Collumbier, MD[b]

[a]Foot and Ankle Department, Hospital for Special Surgery, 523 East 72nd Street,
Suite 514, New York, NY 10021, USA
[b]Clinique de l'Union, Boulevard de Ratalens, BP 24336, Saint Jean, 31240 L'Union Cedex,
Toulouse, France

Although dancers put a great deal of stress through the first metatarsophalangeal joint (MTPJ), it is unlikely that dancing causes bunions. Dancers, like the rest of the population, are either prone to bunions or not [1]. In dancers who have a painful bunion, it is best to employ conservative measures rather than surgical intervention. Any surgery on the first MTPJ will adversely affect dorsiflexion of this joint, which is a critical motion for dancers.

DEVELOPMENT OF BUNIONS IN DANCERS
In ballet, maintaining the "en pointe" stance forces the foot into abduction and increases the relative valgus force on the first MTPJ. Furthermore, forcing a turnout or "rolling in" leads to pronation of the foot with abduction of the hallux and an increase valgus force on the joint. These forces may produce an environment in which dancers may develop bunions.

Two types of bunions are commonly seen in dancers. The first type, slowly progressive bunions, has a normal range of motion secondary to a congruous MTPJ. These dancers are best treated with conservative modalities including pads, ballet shoe stretching, and anti-inflammatory medication when symptomatic. The second type, rapidly progressive bunions, is less common. The dancer is affected by the loss of motion within the joint and has progressive pain. Initially, these painful deformities should be treated conservatively, but surgical intervention is likely to be required as symptoms worsen.

Slowly Progressive Bunions
In these bunions, the joint is generally congruous (Fig. 1). Although often associated with a larger metatarsal head, the congruency of the joint allows the motion of the MTPJ to be maintained. In a ballet dancer, it is not uncommon to see 80° to 90° of dorsiflexion with no joint pain despite an obvious clinical bunion and inflamed bursa.

*Corresponding author. E-mail address: kennedyj@hss.edu (J.G. Kennedy).

0278-5919/08/$ – see front matter
doi:10.1016/j.csm.2007.12.004

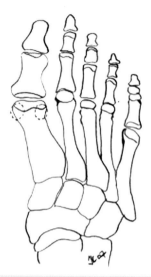

Fig. 1. Congruent bunion. Line drawing with the intermetatarsal angle less than 15° and the first MTPJ articulation congruent. Sesamoid bone is covered by the metatarsal head.

Due to the joint congruity, the sesamoid sling is maintained in an anatomic position, resulting in normal articular mechanics; thus, sesamoid pain is rare in these slowly progressive bunions. This inherent joint stability is reflected radiographically—at least 50% of the sesamoid is covered by the first MT head (see Fig. 1). Other radiographic parameters include an intermetatarsal angle of 11° or less in addition to a hallux valgus angle of 20° or less.

Conservative treatment of slowly progressive bunions includes orthopedic felt or lamb's wool for padding within the ballet slipper when the dancer has symptomatic bursitis. In the case of compression of the superficial dorsal cutaneous nerve, dorsal padding with mole skin or lamb's wool is beneficial. In cases of recalcitrant neuralgia, a short course of pregabalin is used for 5 days to reduce neuropathic symptoms. Horseshoe- and doughnut-shaped pads may be created individually for each dancer and placed within the ballet slipper without compromising the motion of the foot or shoe.

The dancer may also stretch the Achilles tendon two to three times a day for 15 minutes in an effort to reduce forefoot overload in normal gait. No form of brace or night splint has been found to be effective in these slowly progressive bunions. Surgery is generally not required and is best held in reserve until the end of the dancer's career. When surgery is considered in this group of patients, the Chevron osteotomy (Figs. 2 and 3) combined with a Maestro modification of the Aiken procedure will produce the most reproducible results [2–4].

This procedure can be performed through a small incision and is inherently stable, affording rapid return to practice within 8 weeks. A toe spacer should be worn for 3 months to prevent stretch out of the medial capsular repair. The

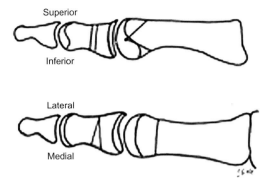

Fig. 2. Chevron osteotomy showing sagittal and anteroposterior) planes. Apex of Chevron is at the center of the head. Dorsal cut can be longer to improve stability. Akin osteotomy of proximal phalanx shows wedge cut to address interphalangeus.

Maestro modification of the Aiken procedure facilitates derotational alignment and valgus realignment of any hallux interphalangeus. In addition, a small dorsal closing wedge may be added to the Aiken procedure to facilitate maximal postoperative dorsiflexion. The authors do not combine the distal metatarsal Chevron osteotomy with a lateral release in the ballet dancer. The additional soft tissue dissection on the lateral side may lead to scarring and reduced postoperative motion. A medial exostectomy and a bursectomy are routinely included in the Chevron procedure. Patients typically spend 2 weeks heel weight bearing and 2 weeks advancing to full weight bearing. At 6 weeks, the dancer may get back to training; however, a toe spacer and strapping may be required for 3 months following surgery. The authors have also abandoned the use of subcuticular monacryl sutures to close these wounds. Irritation at the ends of the wounds where the initial suture and ending suture knot were tied produced small subcuticular abscesses possibly from constant irritation within the dance slipper. Simple 4-0 nylon is used to close the wound

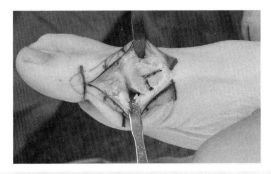

Fig. 3. Intraoperative image of Chevron osteotomy.

and removed at 10 to 14 days following surgery. Few wound complications are encountered using nylon.

Rapidly Progressive Bunions

With rapidly progressive bunions, the dancer generally complains of rapidly increasing deformity associated with pain from an incongruous joint (Fig. 4).

The sesamoid sling is decompensated, with the fibular sesamoid subluxed by over 50% in relation to the first metatarsal head on a plain standing anteroposterior radiograph. This imbalance typically causes the toe to pronate, producing additional tension within the adductor tendon and a laterally deviated great toe. As the hallux moves laterally, the abductor hallucis tendon moves to a more plantar position, acting as a flexor of the MTPJ. The adductor hallucis is now unopposed and has a functionally long lever arm, producing greater deformity. As the valgus angle increases beyond 32°, the push-off power decreases and the dancer begins to shift weight laterally, causing excess loading of the second and third metatarsal [5]. This excess loading may lead to metatarsalgia or stress fractures of the lesser metatarsals. The radiographic picture typically demonstrates a hallux valgus angle greater than 25° with an intermetatarsal angle greater than 12°. These dancers are best treated with conservative measures initially, including mole skin padding and anti-inflammatory medication. Ultimately, the pain will prevent the dancer from performing at a high standard and surgery should be considered.

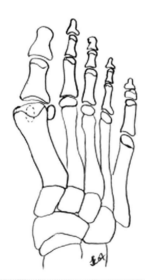

Fig. 4. Incongruent bunion. Line drawing with the intermetatarsal angle greater than 15°. First MTPJ articulation is incongruent. Fibular sesamoid is uncovered, demonstrating luxation of sesamoid sling.

In dancers in whom surgery is considered, the authors use the Scarf osteotomy in conjunction with a modified McBride and Akin proximal phalangeal osteotomy (Figs. 5 and 6).

In this procedure, low-profile screws are used to hold the osteotomy in place. As the construct confers mechanical stability, early motion and weight bearing can be encouraged. In general, the dancer is allowed to exercise using a bicycle for the first 3 weeks following surgery. Swimming is allowed at 3 weeks following surgery, and the dancer may be fully weight bearing doing gentle floor exercises at 8 weeks. Dancers must wear a toe spacer for a period of 3 months, and although general training and conditioning can start at 8 weeks following surgery, no dance maneuvers are allowed until at least 3 months following surgery.

The authors have operated on several elite dancers and have found the SCARF osteotomy to be a useful and reproducible procedure; however, in dancers, it is best to avoid overaggressive rotational translation of the SCARF osteotomy because this can alter the mechanics of the sesamoid sling and produce stiffness within the joint. Although this stiffness can be treated with a joint injection and manipulation, the high demands placed on the first MTPJ by dancers may accelerate arthrosis within the malaligned sesamoid metatarsal joint.

ARTHRITIC BUNIONS

Dancers who have mild arthrosis and loss of cartilage on the head of the first MTPJ visualized at the time of surgery can be treated with a cheilectomy of the dorsal osteophyte and dorsal 25% of the joint as an adjunct to the Chevron or the SCARF osteotomy. To offload the remaining cartilage, care must be taken to release the plantar plate to maximize postoperative motion.

Although it was not described initially as a treatment modality for an arthritic bunion, interpositional arthroplasty (Fig. 7) has been described as an effective method of preserving motion in a severely arthritic first MTPJ [6,7]. In certain cases, the authors use an interpositional graft in a dancer who has an arthritic bunion. In this situation, the metatarsal itself is not osteotomized other

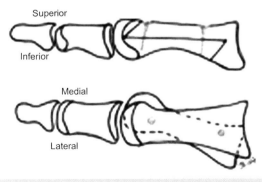

Fig. 5. SCARF osteotomy showing Z-shaped cuts and translational movement and rotation to achieve desired intermetatarsal angle.

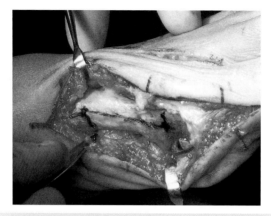

Fig. 6. Intraoperative image of SCARF osteotomy.

than with a standard cheilectomy and medial exostectomy. No realignment osteotomy is performed on the metatarsal; however, a combination of dorsal closing wedge and medial closing wedge osteotomy, the so-called "Maiken," is performed on the proximal phalanx. A single 0.62 Kirschner wire is used to hold the construct in place for 3 weeks following surgery. Following pin removal, the dancer can begin passive and active assisted range of motion of

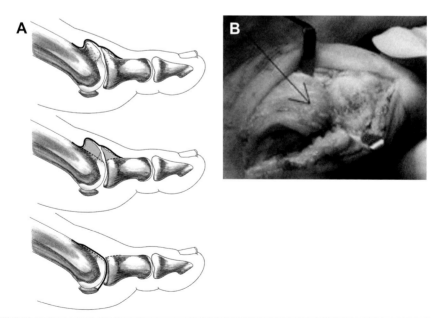

Fig. 7. (A) Interpositional arthroplasty of the first MTPJ. (B) Intraoperative photograph of an interpositional graft in situ; note the capsular graft (arrow).

the joint. At 6 weeks following surgery, the dancer is allowed to begin rehearsal. This mode of treatment allows an early return of painless function in a subset of dancers for whom the only other alternative is retirement.

SECONDARY PROBLEMS ARISING FROM BUNIONS

Metatarsalgia

Because the push-off power of the first MTPJ is reduced as a secondary effect from the progressive deformity of a bunion, weight is transferred to the lesser metatarsal heads. Pain from overload of the lesser metatarsal heads can be more debilitating than a bunion. Treatment is directed at offloading the affected bony prominence and distributing the load using a metatarsal pad. Surgery should be considered only at the end of a dancer's career because any procedure cannot address the metatarsal alone and must consider the tarsometatarsal joint and the adjacent metatarsals. The consequences of such surgery, even when successful, can be career ending.

Stress Fractures

When the foot is pronated secondary to the progressive bunion, abnormal mechanical loads are transferred to the lateral or lesser metatarsal bones and to the lateral aspect of the ankle joint and fibula. A relative metabolic imbalance in bone resorption and production may manifest as a stress fracture, particularly in the second and third metatarsals and occasionally in the lateral fibula. The authors always perform a metabolic profile on the dancer in the presence of a stress fracture to rule out any underlying cause. The dreaded "dancer's triad" must always be considered, and a careful history of diet and nutrition must be taken from all dancers. The treatment is based on addressing the mechanical overload and any metabolic deficiency. A longitudinal arch-support orthotic can help address overpronation, and the dancer may use an ultrasound bone stimulator for a period of 3 weeks to accelerate bone healing. Throughout this 3-week period, the dancer must rest in a cam shoe or boot. Barefoot dancing should be discouraged in those prone to stress fractures.

Sesamoiditis

In a typical decompensated bunion, the sesamoid sling subluxes and the sesamoid metatarsal joint becomes incongruent. As a result, inflammation of the articulating cartilage can cause pain and further degeneration. A dancer's pad or U-shaped pad is usually sufficient to alleviate symptoms. Occasionally, an injection of 10 mg of triamcinolone can be administered into the joint itself. This procedure is best done under ultrasound guidance to facilitate precise positioning and to avoid inadvertent injection of the flexor hallucis brevis.

Flexor Hallucis Longus Tendonitis

Occasionally, the pronated foot, in the presence of a hypermobile first ray, causes the flexor hallucis longus to plantar flex the great hallux to accommodate the first-ray deformity. With prolonged contraction of the great toe long flexor, inflammation may occur. Simple stretching of the toe combined with a semirigid Morton's extension orthotic can alleviate the spasm within the muscle tendon unit.

AVOIDING BUNIONS

Because bunion surgery should be avoided whenever possible in dances of all ages, it is imperative that young dancers learn correct technique. Proper technique may prevent excessive loads on the first MTPJ, which in turn may reduce the incidence of bunions. "Winging" refers to a technique fault in which the feet are forced outward from the ankles toward the fifth toe in a winged fashion. A small degree of "winging" can add to the aesthetic alignment of the line of the leg. In the winged position, an excess of pressure is applied through the first toe, particularly in a pronated foot. This excess pressure can produce an inflammatory synovitis and resultant bunion over time. The dance student should concentrate on placing the center of the foot in line with the midpoint of the ankle and leg, thus avoiding winging and potential bunions. This alignment is particularly important for tendus, relevés, and jumps. Rolling in, or "sickling," can also produce excessive stress through the first MTPJ, resulting in bunion deformity over time.

Practicing relevés with a tennis ball placed between the ankles, with the legs and feet parallel, can help prevent young dancers from developing poor techniques that may produce bunion deformity.

SUMMARY

Symptomatic bunions in the elite dancer present a challenge to the orthopaedic surgeon. All attempts should be made to manage this pathology with conservative treatment. Unfortunately this approach will be unsuccessful in many. Surgical correction, even at best, can force a dancer into early retirement from the elite level and therefore must be approached cautiously and methodically.

References

[1] Einarsdottir H, Troell S, Wykman A. Hallux valgus in ballet dancers: a myth? Foot Ankle Int 1995;16:92–4.
[2] Johnson KA, Cofield RH, Morrey BF. Chevron osteotomy for hallux valgus. Clin Orthop Relat Res 1979;142:44–7.
[3] Lillich JS, Baxter DE. Bunionectomies and related surgery in the elite female middle-distance and marathon runner. Am J Sports Med 1986;14:491–3.
[4] Mitchell LA, Baxter DE. A chevron-Akin double osteotomy for correction of hallux valgus. Foot Ankle 1991;12:7–14.
[5] Yamamoto H, Muneta T, Asahina S, et al. Forefoot pressures during walking in feet afflicted with hallux valgus. Clin Orthop Relat Res 1996;323:247–53.
[6] Hamilton WG, O'Malley MJ, Thompson FM, et al. Roger Mann award 1995. Capsular interposition arthroplasty for severe hallux rigidus. Foot Ankle Int 1997;18:68–70.
[7] Kennedy JG, Chow FY, Dines J, et al. Outcomes after interposition arthroplasty for treatment of hallux rigidus. Clin Orthop Relat Res 2006;445:210–5.

Clin Sports Med 27 (2008) 329–334

CLINICS IN SPORTS MEDICINE

ELSEVIER
SAUNDERS

Nerve Disorders in Dancers

John G. Kennedy, MD, MMSc, MCh, FRCSI, FRCS (Orth)[a,*],
Donald E. Baxter, MD[b]

[a]Foot and Ankle Department, Hospital for Special Surgery, 523 East 72nd Street,
Suite 514, New York, NY 10021, USA
[b]Department of Orthopedic Surgery, Baylor College of Medicine, 2500 Fondren Road,
Suite 350, Houston, TX 77063, USA

D ancers are required to perform at the extreme of physiologic and functional limits. Under such conditions, peripheral nerves are prone to compression. It can often be a challenge for the dancer and the surgeon to identify these nerve complaints when the patient is in the office. The dancer may need to demonstrate the provocative position or use the appropriate footwear to re-create the symptoms before a clinical diagnosis can be made. Electromyographic (EMG) studies, nerve conduction studies, MRI, and ultrasound imaging are useful adjuncts in the diagnosis of these nerve disorders; however, the most reproducible and reliable method of diagnosis remains a careful history and clinical examination.

INTERDIGITAL NEUROMAS

The anatomy of the interdigital nerve complex predisposes the third web space to be anatomically prone to develop symptoms from neuromas. In dancers who are overloading the forefoot in relevé, tendu, or en pointe, the interdigital nerve is compressed by the tight intermetatarsal ligament and the surrounding metatarsals. This compression typically manifests as neuritic pain in the third web space but may also be seen in the adjacent spaces. The dance doctor must rule out proximal nerve pathology from a spinal radiculopathy or dysraphism, especially in a child dancer. Adolescent female dancers should be screened for metabolic disorders and the possibility of lesser metatarsal stress fractures that may mimic neuromas. Second metatarsophalangeal joint capsulitis may also present in a similar fashion to a neuroma and is more common in dancers than a second web space neuroma. Gentle traction on the digit with flexion on the joint can elicit pain within the joint, which is pathognomonic for capsulitis rather than neuritic pain. Mulder's click is a rare and unreliable sign in dancers who have neuromas [1].

*Corresponding author. E-mail address: kennedyj@hss.edu (J.G. Kennedy).

0278-5919/08/$ – see front matter
doi:10.1016/j.csm.2008.01.001
sportsmed.theclinics.com

Treatment should initially address the mechanical overload of the metatarsals, which can be achieved with a 0.25-inch metatarsal pad just proximal to the head of the metatarsal and with wider dance shoes that prevent intermetatarsal crowding. In the dancer who pronates and "sickles," producing excess stress on the lateral rays, a simple orthotic can realign the foot, offloading the lateral aspect.

Corticosteroid injections are frequently used to address neuromas within the foot but should be used judiciously. Because overuse can cause atrophy of the plantar fat pad and degeneration of the collateral ligament or volar plate, the authors typically use ultrasound-guided injection rather than blind injection, with better and more prolonged clinical results [2].

Surgery is reserved for patients who have failed three ultrasound-guided injections. Typically, the intermetatarsal ligament is left intact in dancers to prevent the feet from splaying through the forefoot on elevation. The dancer can return to training in ballet shoes at 3 weeks following surgery and must wear a tight compressive dressing for 6 weeks following surgical excision.

TARSAL TUNNEL SYNDROME

The tarsal tunnel is composed of the flexor retinaculum, the medial malleolus, the talus, the medial wall of the calcaneus, and the distal tibia. It contains the long flexor tendons and the posterior tibial artery and vein. The canal also contains the tibial nerve and its branches (Fig. 1).

The calcaneal nerve is the most proximal and most posterior of all branches. The first branch of the lateral plantar nerve courses into a myofascial tunnel within the substance of the abductor hallucis. In ballet dancers, the tunnel may be compressed by a hypertrophic muscle of the flexor hallucis longus, and dancers typically experience dysesthesia on the plantar surface of the foot in relevé [3,4].

The site of the compression—at a point proximal to the tarsal tunnel at the level of the lower fibers of the gastrocnemius muscle, at the tunnel itself, or at the point of the first branch of the lateral plantar nerve as it enters the fascia within the abductor hallucis—can be tested manually with a nerve compression test. In patients in whom clinical examination is equivocal, nerve conduction studies and EMG may be performed. Because these tests are often negative, the senior author prefers that the dancer produce provocative maneuvers that reproduce the symptoms. Under ultrasound guidance, a diagnostic local anesthestic can then be administered. After the diagnosis is made, conservative therapy is initially the best mode of treatment. In dancers who have a high tarsal tunnel, therapy is initially indicated to break the cycle of inflammation, with iontophoresis followed by stretching exercises of the gastrocnemius-soleus complex. A longitudinal ach support may also help by inverting the foot and relieving pressure over the medial column. When surgery is indicated following failure of conservative therapy, nerve dissection is best kept to a minimum. In this way, residual dysesthesia is reduced. The dancer is generally encouraged to bear weight on the affected foot at 7 to 10 days following surgery. Earlier weight bearing can result in bleeding and subsequent scarring that can cause

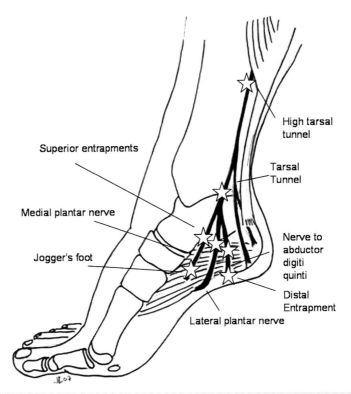

Fig. 1. Areas of compression of the posterior tibial nerve and its branches.

prolonged recovery. In many dancers, the urge to get back rehearsal following surgery is overzealous. In such instances, the senior author places the dancer's foot and ankle in a cast for 2 weeks until the risk has been reduced. At 1 month following surgery, the dancer may resume light training but should be warned that symptoms may last for up to 6 months.

MEDIAL HALLUCAL NERVE

Pain under the tibial sesamoid in dancers may indicate a compression of the medial hallucal nerve as it exits the abductor hallucis muscle fascia (ie, Joplin's neuroma) [5,6]. This condition may often be confused with sesamoiditis. In general, a nerve compression test just proximal to the sesamoid elicits a positive response. A small local anesthetic administered to this area generally confirms the diagnosis. Treatment is usually conservative, with a dancers pad or dough-nut lamb's wool pad within the dance slipper. In recalcitrant cases, surgical re-lease may be performed using a medial incision, avoiding the plantar skin.

ANTERIOR TARSAL TUNNEL SYNDROME

The deep peroneal nerve runs between the extensor digitorum longus and the extensor hallucis longus 5 cm above the ankle mortice. Approximately 1 cm above the ankle joint, under the extensor retinaculum, the nerve divides into a medial and lateral nerve. The medial branch continues with the dorsalis pedis artery under the inferior extensor retinaculum, where it may become compressed by tight ribbon tying patterns over the talonavicular joint [7,8].

Dysesthesia in the first web space is an indicator of compression of the medial branch of the deep peroneal nerve. The lateral branch of the deep peroneal nerve (Fig. 2) divides approximately 1 cm above the ankle mortice. The nerve sends sensory branches to the ankle joint that are critical in maintaining functional ankle stability. The nerve also sends sensory fibers to the roof of the sinus tarsi and travels in a fibrous tunnel beneath the extensor digitorum brevis to supply this muscle with motor function. In this area, the nerve can be compressed over the head of the talus, particularly when the ankle is in a plantarflexed position and inverted [9].

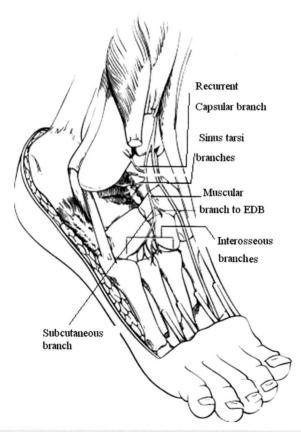

Fig. 2. The lateral branch of the deep peroneal nerve and its branches.

Patients typically present with dorsal foot pain radiating to the lateral Lisfranc's joints in the case of compression of the lateral branch of the deep peroneal nerve. In patients who have medial nerve entrapment, the symptoms are typically within the first web space.

Examination of the dancer should include a thorough evaluation of the deep peroneal nerve as it courses from behind the neck of the fibula. In some patietns, the symptoms of deep peroneal nerve entrapment are brought on by an exertional compartment pressure increase within the anterior compartment.

The precise site of compression is best confirmed with a local nerve block. Surgical release is reserved for recalcitrant cases and should be very site specific to reduce scarring from extensive nerve dissection.

SUPERFICIAL PERONEAL NERVE

The superficial peroneal nerve branches from the common peroneal nerve and courses through the anterolateral compartment of the leg, innervating the peroneus longus and brevis. About one hands' breadth above the ankle joint or 10 to 13 cm above the tip of the lateral malleolus, the nerve pierces the deep fascia of the leg and becomes subcutaneous. At this point, the nerve divides further into two subcutaneous branches, the intermediate and medial dorsal cutaneous nerves [10].

As the nerve pierces the deep fascia, it may become entrapped. This situation is typically seen in dancers who have sickling and eversion of the ankle joint and hypertrophic peroneal musculature. In such cases, a local compartment pressure increase may cause entrapment of the nerve in a short fibrous tunnel [11].

In dancers in whom there is a lateral ligament deficiency or functional ankle instability, the superficial peroneal nerve may be stretched, and any tethering of the nerve as it emerges from the deep compartment to the superficial compartment may predispose to dysesthesia. Most dancers complain of lateral leg pain at the junction of the distal one third and proximal two thirds of the leg. The pain is precipitated by dancing and relieved by rest. Dysesthesia may be elicited in the dorsum and lateral aspect of the foot. The symptoms may be elicited by everting the foot, by dorsiflexing the ankle, and by tapping over the nerve as it emerges from the deep fascia. Care must be taken to avoid confusing these symptoms from those of the lateral branch of the deep peroneal nerve.

Treatment is initially directed at treating the cause. If a ballet shoe ribbon is tied at the exit of the nerve, then its placement needs to be altered. If the ankle is unstable, then functional and mechanical stability training is encouraged. Stretch on the nerve can be reduced by avoiding any excess varus or valgus hindfoot positioning. Surgery is rarely required; however, in such cases, a simple decompression of the fascia around the nerve exit point is all that is needed. The dancer can resume normal practice at 3 weeks after decompression.

SURAL NERVE ENTRAPMENT

The sural nerve runs between the two heads of the gastrocnemius muscle. It travels down the leg along the lateral border of the Achilles tendon, along with the short saphenous vein. Approximately 2 cm above the ankle joint, the nerve divides into a lateral branch that supplies sensation to the lateral heel and a branch that runs plantar to the peroneal sheath, where it then branches to cutaneous nerves supplying the fifth toe and fourth web space. The nerve is rarely injured in ballet or dance. Occasionally, a neurapraxia can be seen in cases of extreme ankle instability, whereby the nerve is compressed by the fifth metatarsal, compressive shoe wear, and an inverted foot. Local measures, such as the use of a small lateral heel pad, are usually sufficient to alleviate the symptoms.

SUMMARY

Entrapment neuropathies in dance can be related to the sciatic nerve or from a radiculopathy related to posture or a hyperlordosis. When a dancer presents with foot and ankle dysesthesia, it is mandatory to examine the back and higher centers to rule out other causes. When the dysesthesia is caused by local nerve compression or irritation, the cause is generally treated with conservative measures, addressing the mechanical balance of the ankle or altering performance footwear and dance surfaces. Surgery is rarely indicated but when it is, consideration must be made to minimize nerve handling to avoid cicatrization and prolonged recovery times.

References

[1] Mulder JD. The causative mechanism in Morton's metatarsalgia. J Bone Joint Surg Br 1951;33:94–5.

[2] Adler RS, Sofka CM. Percutaneous ultrasound-guided injections in the musculoskeletal system. Ultrasound Q 2003;19:3–12.

[3] Baxter DE, Thigpen CM. Heel pain—operative results. Foot Ankle 1984;5:16–25.

[4] Baxter DE, Pfeffer GB. Treatment of chronic heel pain by surgical release of the first branch of the lateral plantar nerve. Clin Orthop Relat Res 1992;279:229–36.

[5] Joplin RJ. The proper digital nerve, vitallium stem arthroplasty, and some thoughts about foot surgery in general. Clin Orthop Relat Res 1971;76:199–212.

[6] Still GP, Fowler MB. Joplin's neuroma or compression neuropathy of the plantar proper digital nerve to the hallux: clinicopathologic study of three cases. J Foot Ankle Surg 1998;37:524–30.

[7] Kopell HP, Thompson WA. Peripheral entrapment neuropathies of the lower extremity. N Engl J Med 1960;262:56–60.

[8] Mackey D, Colbert DS, Chater EH. Musculo-cutaneous nerve entrapment. Ir J Med Sci 1977;146:100–2.

[9] Kennedy JG, Brunner JB, Bohne WH, et al. Clinical importance of the lateral branch of the deep peroneal nerve. Clin Orthop Relat Res 2007;459:222–8.

[10] Saraffian SK. Anatomy of the foot and ankle: descriptive, topographical, functional. Philadelphia: Lippincott; 1983.

[11] Styf J. Entrapment of the superficial peroneal nerve: diagnosis and results of decompression. J Bone Joint Surg Br 1989;71:131–5.

Clin Sports Med 27 (2008) 335–338

CLINICS IN SPORTS MEDICINE

ELSEVIER
SAUNDERS

INDEX

A

Achilles tendon, acute tendinitis of, 281, 282
  anatomy of, 281
  degenerated, 281, 282, 283
  injury of, factors contributing to, 281
  of foot, 285–286
  rupture of, 283
  sources pf pain in, 281
  stretching of, in bunions, 322

Achilles tendonitis, initial treatment
  of, 281–282

Achilles tendonosis, 282–283

Ankle, and foot, injuries in dancers, incidence
  of, 247–248
  and foot fractures, generic treatment
    strategy for, 296
    in dancers, **295–304**
      assessment of, 296
      clinical presentation of, 296
      factors contributing to, 295
  and foot injuries, level of, predictors of,
    295–296
  Baker's cyst of, 266
  injuries of, etiology and biomechanics
    of, 248
  instability of, chronic, definition of, 257
    surgery in, 258–259
    treatment of, 258–259
    types of, 258
    combined, 258
    dance-specific risk factors for,
      249–251
    functional, 258
    mechanical, 258
    risk factors for, 248–251
    sprains and, in dancers, **247–262**
  lateral injury of, 251–253
    grading of, 252
    presentation and assessment
      of, 252–253
  medial, 290
    injury of, 253
      in osteochrondral lesion
        of talus, 253, 254
    pain in, differential diagnosis
      of, 268, 269

versus posterior pain in, 274
  sprains of, 267–268
    treatment of, 268
  posterior, anatomy of, 263, 264
    pain in, differential diagnosis
      of, 266
      in dancers, **263–277**
        operative treatment
          of, 270–275
        versus medial pain, 274
    pseudomeniscus in, 270
    posterior impingement of, flexor hallucis
      longus tendonitis versus, 273
    posterior impingement syndrome
      of, 268–269
      treatment of, 270
        results of, 275–276
    posterolateral pain in, 268–270
      causes of, 270
    posteromedial pain in, 263–268
    sprains of, acute, recurrence of, 257
      and instability, conservative versus
        surgical treatment of, 257
        in dancers, **247–262**
        incidence of, 247
          in dancers, 248
        lateral, grading of, 252
    stability of, ligaments promoting, 248

Anterior talofibular ligament, 248, 249,
  251–252
  grade I injury (sprain or stretch)
    of, 256
  grade II injury (partial tear) of, 256
  grade III injury of, 256

Anterior tarsal tunnel syndrome, 255,
  331–333

Arhtroplasty procedure, interpositional,
  310, 311

Arthritis bunions, 325–327

Arthroplasty, interpositional, in arthritic
  bunions, 325, 326

B

Baker's cyst of ankle, 266

Blisters, 316

Note: Page numbers of article titles are in **boldface** type.

0278-5919/08/$ – see front matter
doi:10.1016/S0278-5919(08)00017-3

Bunionette, 315, 316
  treatment of, 315–316
Bunions, arthritic, 325
      treatment of, 325–327
  in dancers, **321–328**
      avoiding of, 328
      development of, 321–325
      rapidly progressive, 324
          treatment of, 325, 326
      secondary problems arising from, 327–328
      slowly progressive, 321–322
          treatment of, 322–324

C

Calcanceus, stress fractures of, 297, 298
Calcaneal nerve, 330
Calcaneofibular ligament, 250, 252
  grade III injury, 256
Calluses, 316
Cavus foot, 267
  posterior tibial tendon and, 291
Cheilectomy, in arthritic bunions, 325
Chevron osteotomy, with Maestro modification of Aiken procedure, in bunions, 322–324
Colliculus, fracture of, 268
Corns, 316
Cross-training, 291–292
Cuboid, subluxation of, 255
      physical findings in, 255
      treatment of, 255

D

Dancer's fracture, 300–301
  of fifth metatarsal, 318
Dancer's tendinitis, 263–264
Dancer's tendonitis, 285, 291
Dancing en pointe, 249–250, 287
Deltoid ligament, chronic strain of, 253
Demi-pointe position, 250, 251, 287

E

En-pointe position, 249–250, 287
Exercises, range-of-motion, in ankle sprains, 259

F

Female athlete triad, 296, 305
Fibro-osseous tunnel, 263
Fibula, stress fractures of, 297

Flatfoot, and posterior tibial tendon insufficiency, 290
Flexor hallucis longus, 263, 285–286, 290
  anatomy of, 285
  fibrotic torn, 286
  tenolysis of, and excision of os trigonum from medial approach, 271–275
Flexor hallucis longus tendonitis, 265–266, 270, 286
  due to bunion deformity, 327
  versus posterior impingement of ankle, 273
Flexor hallucis longus tenosynovitis, medial pain in, 291
Foot, and ankle, injuries in dancers, incidence of, 247–248
  and ankle fractures, generic treatment strategy for, 296
      in dancers, **295–304**
          assessment of, 296
          clinical presentation of, 296
          factors contributing to, 295
  and ankle injuries, level of, predictors of, 295–296
Footwear, pointe, 251
Forefoot injuries, ballet and, 305
  in acute trauma, 305
  in dancers, **305–320**
Fractures. See specific sites and types of fractures.
Freiberg's infarction, 313–314
Full-pointe position, 249
Fungal infection, of toenails, 306

G

Grand Plié in fifth position, 266, 267
Great toe, 306–313

H

Hallucal nerve, medial, compression of, 331
Hallux rigidus, 308–310
  causes of, 309
  functional, 266
  grading systems for, 309
  pseudo-, 286
  treatment of, 310, 311, 312
Hallux saltans, 264, 265, 286
Hallux valgus, 307–308
Health, good, importance to prevent injury, 305
Hematomas, subungual, 306

I

Ingrown toenails, 306

Interphalangeal joint, fifth proximal, unstable, 315
    hyperflexion injuries of, 307

Inversion injury, associated injuries in, 253–254, 255

J

Jogger's foot, 266

Jones fractures, 301, 302

K

Kinetic chain dysfunctions, in ballet dancers, 248

L

Ligament complex, lateral, 251–252
    injuries of, treatment of, 256–257

M

Mallet toe, 316

Medial malleolus, pain around, 268

Medial prominence, contusion of, 268

Metatarsalgia, due to bunion deformity, 327

Metatarsal(s), fifth, dancer's fracture of, 318
    fractures of, 300–301
    injuries of, 317–318
    second, stress fractures of, 299–300, 317–318

Metatarsophalangeal joint(s), 264
    dislocation of, 315
    first, injuries of, 307–313
    injuries of, 313–315
    instability of, 314–315

Metatarsophalangeal synovitis, idiopathic, 315

N

Nails, condition of, revealing health issues, 306

Navicular stress fractures, 297–298

Nerve disorders, in dancers, **329–334**

Nerve entrapment, mimicking sesamoiditis, 313

Nerve impingement, as cause of post sprain pain, 255

Neuromas, interdigital, 329
    treatment of, 330

O

Oblique spiral shaft fractures, 300–301

Onychocryptosis, 306

Onychomycosis, 306

Os subtibiale, 253, 254, 268

Os trigonum, 263
    ankles with and without, 265, 269
    excision of, 270, 271
        from medial approach, tenolysis of flexor hallucis longus and, 271–275
        using lateral approach, 275
    management of, 270
    posterior impingement syndrome in, 268–269

Osteochrondral autologous transplant surgery, 253, 254

P

Paratenonitis, 280

Paronychia, acute, 306

Peroneal nerve, deep, compression of, 256
    examination of, 256
    lateral branch of, 332
    superficial, entrapment of, 333
        treatment of, 333

Peroneal tendonitis, cuboid dysfunction in, 255
    treatment of, 284

Peroneal tendons, 283–284
    functions of, 284
    longitudinal tears or subluxation of, 254–255
    pathology of, in dancers, 284

Peroneus brevis, incomplete tear of, 284

Phalangeal fractures, 303

Phalangeal stress fractures, 307

Phalanges, and interphalangeal joint, 307

Plantar flexion sign, 269

Pointe shoes, 251

Posterior impingement syndrome, in os trigonum, 268–269
    of ankle, 268–269
        treatment of, 270
            results of, 275–276

Posterior talofibular ligament, 252

Proprioception, in dancers, evaluation of, 257

Pseudomeniscus, in posterior ankel, 270

R

Radiographs, in lateral ankle pain, 252–253

Range-of-motion exercises, in ankle sprains, 259

Retrofibular space, 284

S

SCARF osteotomy, in rapidly progressive bunions, 325, 326

Sesamoid bursitis, 313

Sesamoid instability, 313

Sesamoidectomy, 312

Sesamoiditis, 302, 303, 311
  due to bunion deformity, 327
  treatment of, 311–312

Sesamoids, 301–303
  fracture of, 302, 303
  injuries of, 302, 310–313
    causes of, 310
    differential diagnosis of, 310
    treatment of, 302

Shoes, pointe, 251

Sickling, 308, 318, 328

Stieda's process, 263

Strength training, in ankle sprains, 259

Stress fractures, 297–300
  calcaneal, 297, 298
  due to bunion deformity, 327
  fibular, 297
  medial tibial, 291
  navicular, 297–298
    os navicular and, 298
      treatment of, 299
    sagittal plane, 298
  of proximal fifth metatarsal diaphysis, 300
  of second metatarsal, 299–300, 317–318
  phalangeal, 307

Stress injuries, in repetitive microtrauma, 295

Subungual hematomas, 306

Sural nerve, entrapment of, 334

T

Talar compression syndrome, 268–269
  treatment of, 270
    results of, 275–276

Talofibular ligament, anterior, 248, 249, 251–252
    grade I injury (sprain or stretch) of, 256
    grade II injury (partial tear) of, 256
    grade III injury of, 256
  posterior, 252

Talus, osteochondral lesion of, 253, 254
    treatment of, 253, 254
  posterior process of, 263
  two tubercles of, 263, 264

Tarsal tunnel syndrome, 266, 330–331, 331
  anterior, 255, 331–333
  treatment of, 330–331

Tendinopathy, 280

Tendinosis, 280

Tendonitis, 280

Tendon(s), injuries of, in dance, **279–288**
    terminology associated with, 280
  injury of, etiology of, 280
    examination of dancer with, 280–281
    histologic response to, 280
  structure of, 279
  tears of, 265

Thomasen's sign, 266, 267

Tibial tendinitis, posterior, 267

Tibial tendon, anterior, anatomy of, 286
  posterior, 285, 290
    anatomy of, 289
    biomechanics of, 289
    injury in young athlete, and posterior tibial tendon insufficiency, 290
    insufficiency, and posterior tibial tendon injury to young athlete, 290
    flatfoot and, 290
  repaired, 292, 293
  tear(s) of, case reviews of, 291–293
    diagnosis of, 290–291
    differential diagnosis of, 291
    in dancers, **289–294**

Tibial tendonitis, treatment of, 285

Tibial tendonosis, posterior, 285

Toenails, fungal infection of, 306
  infections of, 306
  ingrown, 306
  injuries to, 306

Toe(s), dislocation of, 303–304
  great, 306–313
  lesser, injuries of, 313–316
    miscellaneous problems of, 313–316
  mallet, 316

Tuberosity fractures, 300

Turnout, in ballet, injuries associated with, 250

W

Winging, 328